Psychosomatic Obstetrics and Gynecology

Advances in Psychosomatic Medicine

Vol. 12

Series Editor
Thomas N. Wise, Falls Church, Va.

Editors
G. Fava, Bologna; *H. Freyberger,* Hannover;
F. Guggenheim, Dallas, Tex.; *O. W. Hill,* London;
Z. J. Lipowski, Toronto; *G. Lloyd,* Edinburgh;
J. C. Nemiah, Boston, Mass.; *A. Reading,* Tampa, Fla.;
P. Reich, Boston, Mass.

Consulting Editors
G. L. Engel, Rochester, N. Y.; *H. Weiner,* Bronx, N. Y.;
L. Levi, Stockholm

Editor Emeritus
Franz Reichsman, Brooklyn, N. Y.

KARGER

S. Karger · Basel · München · Paris · London · New York · Tokyo · Sydney

Psychosomatic Obstetrics and Gynecology

Volume Editors
M. B. Rosenthal, Cleveland, Ohio
D. H. Smith, Cleveland, Ohio

4 figures, 1985

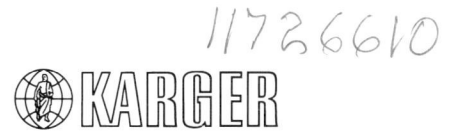

KARGER

S. Karger · Basel · München · Paris · London · New York · Tokyo · Sydney

Advances in Psychosomatic Medicine

National Library of Medicine, Cataloging in Publication
    Psychosomatic obstetrics and gynecology/
    volume editors, M.B. Rosenthal, D.H. Smith.
    — Basel; New York: Karger, 1985. —
    (Advances in psychosomatic medicine; vol. 12)
    Includes index.
    1. Genital Diseases, Female 2. Obstetrics 3. Psychosomatic Medicine I. Rosenthal, M.B. (Miriam B.)
    II. Smith, D.H. (Dennis H.) III. Series
    W1 AD81 v. 12 [WQ 100 P9735]
    ISBN 3–8055–3967–3

Drug Dosage
    The authors and the publisher have exerted every effort to ensure that drug selection and dosage set forth in this text are in accord with current recommendations and practice at the time of publication. However, in view of ongoing research, changes in government regulations, and the constant flow of information relating to drug therapy and drug reactions, the reader is urged to check the package insert for each drug for any change in indications and dosage and for added warnings and precautions. This is particularly important when the recommended agent is a new and/or infrequently employed drug.

All rights reserved.
    No part of this publication may be translated into other languages, reproduced or utilized in any form or by any means, electronic or mechanical, including photocopying, recording, microcopying, or by any information storage and retrieval system, without permission in writing from the publisher.

©   Copyright 1985 by S. Karger AG, P.O. Box, CH-4009 Basel (Switzerland)
    Printed in Switzerland by Merkur Druck AG, Langenthal
    ISBN 3–8055–3967–3

Contents

Smith, D.H.; Rosenthal, M.B. (Cleveland, Ohio): Editorial 1
Schnatz, P.T. (Cleveland, Ohio): Neuroendocrinology and the Ovulation Cycle – Advances and Review. 4
Youngs, D.D. (Portland, Me.); *Reame, N.* (Ann Arbor, Mich.): Psychoendocrinology and the Menstrual Cycle 25
DeFazio, J.; Austin, C.; Speroff, L. (Cleveland, Ohio): Pathophysiologic Basis for the Menopause 35
Lothstein, L.M. (Cleveland, Ohio): Female Sexuality and Feminine Development: Freud and His Legacy 57
Gyves, M.T. (Cleveland, Ohio): The Psychosocial Impact of High Risk Pregnancy 71
Stotland, N.L. (Chicago, Ill.); *Peterson, C.* (Washington, D.C.): A Modest Proposal: Breastfeeding for the Infants of Adolescent Mothers. 81
Stotland, N.L. (Chicago, Ill.): Psychological Implications of Recent Developments in Peripartum Care 91
Small, E.C. (Reno, Nev.); *Turksoy, R.N.* (Boston, Mass.): A View of Artificial Insemination 105
Guzinski, G.M. (Baltimore, Md.): Advances in the Diagnosis and Treatment of Chronic Pelvic Pain 124
Wise, T.N. (Falls Church, Va.): Sexual Dysfunctions following Diseases of the Reproductive Organs 136
Klonoff, E.A.; Janata, J.W. (Cleveland, Ohio): Use of Behavior Therapy in Obstetrics and Gynecology 150
Mahowald, M.B. (Cleveland, Ohio): Obgynethical Issues – Present and Future 166

Subject Index 182

Editorial

Dennis H. Smith, Miriam B. Rosenthal

The changes in obstetrics and gynecology that have occurred since the beginning of the 20th century have been so great as to make this specialty almost unrecognizable to those practitioners who lived in the 19th century. The need for technical expertise and surgical excellence are still required; but the need for an understanding of pathophysiology and psychological mechanisms has greatly increased. Some of the departments of obstetrics and gynecology have in fact changed their names to 'reproductive biology': an attempt to show the inseparability of the basic sciences and clinical practice. With the tremendous explosion of knowledge and techniques in anesthesia, antisepsis and antibiotics, gynecologic surgery expanded not only to prolong life, but to enhance the quality of life. It is awesome to recall that at the present time, women have approximately one-third of their lives to live after the menopause.

The knowledge of endocrinology in reproductive biology has greatly increased. Irregular menstrual cycles, infertility, contraception, and the physiologic effects of the menopause have all become subject to manipulation by the medical practitioner. The emergence of perinatalogy or high-risk obstetrics has enabled more women afflicted with serious medical illnesses to have living children and with neonatology has pushed the age of infant survival to very young gestational ages.

Many of these advances have brought with them a significant threat to the psychological well-being of women. The gynecologist of the past often tended to be paternalistic with little regard to the patient's feelings. The techniques of surgery, especially cancer surgery, sometimes seemed more directed towards the cure of an alien cancer than toward the rehabilitation of a stricken woman. Infertility investigation and treatment tended to reduce lovemaking to a 'by the numbers' process. Long weeks and months of hospitalization on high-risk pregnancy wards remind us of the emotional deprivation once suffered by victims of tuberculosis. The use of monitoring during labor added a mechanical aspect which could be intrusive if not introduced in the proper way to the patient – or used as a substitute for human interaction. The effect of somatic illness and its treatment on the emotional and behavioral aspects of the woman have become increasingly evident. What of the effect of the psyche on the soma?

Psychology is now a basic science essential to the study of reproduction and to the practice of obstetrics and gynecology. The impact of thought, stress, and emotion on the hypothalamus with subsequent alteration of hormonal function is evident in the study of reproductive function. Thus, a complete interdependence of psyche and soma is a fundamental concept. There is evidence that neurotransmitters are involved in affect and perhaps thought. The woman's thoughts and feelings about her femininity come from childhood experiences and the changing world about her, and affect the whole range of reproductive function from childhood through old age.

The changing role of women and men in society, therefore, becomes an important factor in the health care of women. Approximately 50% of the United States work force is now made up of women. The stresses of competing for career goals are increasingly affecting the health of women. Delay in childbearing to an older age increases the chances of obstetrical complications. Breast-feeding and child-rearing must be coordinated with work plans. Thus, marriage has taken on a new aspect of mutual sharing which will sometimes involve expertise in this field from the patient's health provider. The climacteric and menopause bring physiologic stresses and psychologic mid-life adjustments to bear on the woman. Chronic illness and chronic pain may be crippling to some individuals and well tolerated by others. As one reads the chapters of this volume, it becomes increasingly clear that those health personnel who treat women must be aware of physiologic and psychologic factors. The complete interdependence of psyche and soma necessitates a psychosomatic approach to obstetrics and gynecology.

This volume covers a number of issues important in the field of psychosomatic obstetrics and gynecology. It starts with an overview by Dr. *Schnatz* of the neuroendocrinology of the ovulation cycle and basic concepts that are essential to understanding reproduction. Dr. *Youngs,* a specialist in both obstetrics and gynecology and psychiatry, and Dr. *Reame* then discuss the psychosomatic consideration of menstrual disorders.

Continuing the basic foundations in new advances in pathophysiology, a team of gynecological endocrinologists, Drs. *DeFazio, Austin,* and *Speroff,* discuss the menopause. Dr. *Lothstein,* a psychologist, then presents the psychology of female sexuality and feminine development. Dr. *Gyves,* a perinatologist, describes issues involved in high-risk pregnancy. The emotional aspects of breast-feeding and perinatal care are presented by Drs. *Stotland* and *Peterson.* Artificial insemination and its relation to infertility are considered by Drs. *Small* and *Turksoy.* The difficulties facing chronic pain patients and some ways to help them are explained by Dr. *Guzinski,* a gynecologist. Dr. *Wise,* a psychiatrist, discusses the phenomenon of sexual dysfunction following diseases of reproductive organs. Behavioral treatment in reproductive system problems is presented by a psychologist, Dr. *Klonoff,* and Dr. *Janata.* A philosopher, Dr. *Mahowald,* presents a final chapter on bioethics in obstetrics and gynecology. This chapter challenges each practitioner of obstetrics and gynecology to look at his or her own ethical systems as well as those of the patients in an effort to best practice obstetrics and gynecology in a manner that considers the whole patient: the patient as a physician-scientist sees her, the patient as the psychologist sees her, and perhaps as important or more important, as the patient sees herself.

Neuroendocrinology and the Ovulation Cycle – Advances and Review

Paul T. Schnatz

Department of Reproductive Biology, Case Western Reserve University School of Medicine; Division of Reproductive Endocrinology and Infertility, University Hospitals, Cleveland, Ohio, USA

The science of neuroendocrinology has advanced dramatically in the last decade and a half. Transplantation and pituitary stalk section experiments [21] established the concept that chemical substances from the brain have an effect on the synthesis and release of pituitary trophic hormones. Early experiments involved the use of extracts from the rodent hypothalamus and demonstrated that hypothalamic extracts could produce changes in the circulating levels of gonadotropins. Much of the early work was done with bioassays and it was difficult to measure a specific endpoint. As radioimmunoassays for protein and steroid hormones were developed, it became easier to determine the effect of hypothalamic substances on pituitary gonadotropin secretion. Eventually the specific chemical structure was identified for thyrotropin-releasing hormone (TRH) and luteinizing hormone-releasing hormone (LH-RH) or gonadotropin-releasing hormone (GnRH) as it has now come to be known. For this work *Guillemin* [12] and *Schally* [32] were awarded the Nobel Prizes in 1977. With chemical identification and synthesis of releasing hormones, it has been possible to develop a basic understanding of the complex relationships between hypothalamus, pituitary, and ovary.

It is now apparent that the hypothalamus supplies several types of chemical signals to the pituitary which are both stimulatory and inhibitory. These signals seem to be separate for each pituitary trophic hormone although there is considerable overlap. It has not been possible yet to identify both stimulating and inhibiting hypothalamic factors or hormones for all pituitary hormones. An example of this is prolactin for which no specific releasing factor has been identified. Prolactin secretion is controlled by prolactin-inhibiting factor (PIF) which is believed by most to be dopamine. It is true that TRH causes increases of pituitary prolactin secretion but it is not believed that TRH is part of the normal physiologic regulatory system for prolactin [29].

The system is one in which chemical substances from the hypothalamus act on the pituitary to stimulate and inhibit pituitary hormone secretion. These substances are transported from the hypothalamus to the anterior pituitary via a portal system of vessels. The hypothalamic releasing factors and hormones are modified by biogenic amines, catecholamines, endogenous opiates, catecholestrogens, and probably several other factors. Many of the modifying factors are affected by external and environmental factors. Regular, normal menses occur only when the hypothalamus, pituitary and ovary are functioning in a coordinated manner. It is no wonder that chronic disease, change in emotional state, stress, medication, and a host of other internal and external factors can significantly affect the normal functioning of the ovulation cycle. The purpose of this chapter is to review the normal ovulation cycle and the hormonal events which lead to ovulation, corpus luteum formation, and pregnancy if fertilization occurs. Recent concepts of neuroendocrinology will be discussed as they relate to the ovulation cycle.

The Normal Ovulation Cycle

The human ovulation cycle involves a series of interrelated events which occur simultaneously at several different levels. Regular cyclic bleeding accompanied by menstrual molimina is an indication that estrogen and progesterone are being produced in a normal organized manner and are having an effect on the endometrium as well as other target organs. The secretion of ovarian hormones is regulated in part by pituitary gonadotropins and modified by feedback mechanisms. Hypothalamic gonadotropin releasing hormone (GnRH) secreted in a pulsatile fashion is necessary to achieve appropriate and coordinated secretion of pituitary gonadotropins. A change of hormone environment at any level of the system can change target organ sensitivity, affect hormone secretion at other levels, and produce abnormalities in the system. The most obvious manifestations of changes are abnormalities of bleeding.

The ovulation cycle as a whole is the result of three factors: 1) the organization of the follicle which permits it to grow and secrete estrogen in an exponential fashion, 2) the constant stimulus to the follicle by FSH and LH, and 3) the organization of the hypothalamic-pituitary system which allows the pituitary to produce a surge of LH in response to a critical level of estrogen secreted by the follicle and in response to its exposure to GnRH. The other elements of the cycle such as ovulation, corpus luteum formation, secretion of estrogen and progesterone and their effects on the reproductive tract follow from these three elements.

Summary of the Principal Events
Which Occur during the Human Ovulation Cycle

Figure 1 is a summary of the main hormonal events which occur during the ovulation cycle. Note that the hormone levels are presented as percent of maximum secretion rather than specific values. There is a slow rise of estrogen during the first half of the follicular phase of the cycle with a rapid exponential rise before the midcycle LH surge which always precedes ovulation. The second peak of estrogen occurs during the luteal phase and is primarily from the corpus luteum. Progesterone secretion is very low during the follicular phase with an approximate 2-fold rise during and immediately preceding ovulation and then a marked rise during the period of active corpus luteum secretion. Estrogen and progesterone normally decrease 2–3 days before the onset of bleeding. This decrease allows an increase of follicle-stimulating hormone (FSH) which stimulates follicle growth and estrogen secretion. As estrogen increases, FSH slowly decreases because of the inhibitory effect of estrogen on FSH. LH is also slightly decreased by rising estrogen levels but not as dramatically as FSH. When a certain level of estrogen (300–500 pg/ml) is reached for a specific period of time (36–48 h), estrogen has a positive stimulatory effect on LH resulting in the LH surge which precedes ovulation by approximately 16–30 h. The stimulatory effect of estrogen on LH is due, at least in part, to an increased sensitivity of the pituitary to pulses of GnRH. During the luteal phase of the cycle, both FSH and LH are depressed because of the synergistic effect of estrogen and progesterone in decreasing the secretion of pituitary gonadotropins. This is probably mediated through a change in pituitary sensitivity to GnRH but could involve other mechanisms.

Oogenesis and Follicle Formation

Oogonia are derived either from primordial germ cells or from celomic epithelium covering the genital ridges and they multiply by mitosis during

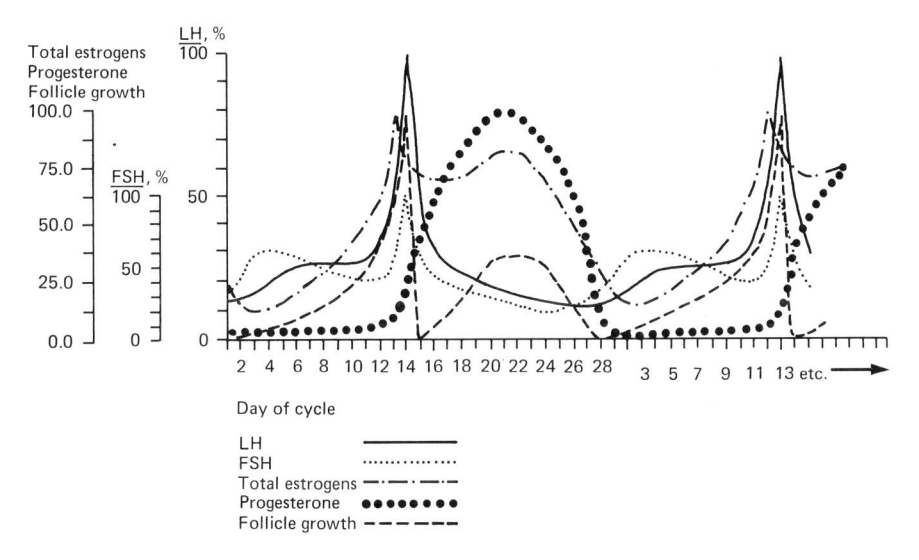

Fig. 1. Summary of hormonal events – normal ovulation cycle. Hormone levels are presented as percent maximum secretion.

embryogenesis. When mitosis stops before birth, the first of two meiotic divisions starts and stops in prophase. No further division occurs until ovulation. At this point the oogonium is referred to as a primary oocyte and once it has been surrounded by a single layer of flattened epithelial cells (pregranulosa cells), the unit thus formed is called a primordial follicle. The primordial follicles represent a pool of follicle units which are located in the ovarian cortex and are ready to grow and develop when given the proper stimulation. The number of follicle units is highest at about 20 weeks of gestation (6–7 million) and decreases continuously so that about a million are present at birth, and by age 50, nearly all the primordial follicles are gone. The decrease in number is due to the process of atresia. Once the number of follicle units in the ovary reaches a critically low level, the ovulation cycle ceases. The usual age at which this occurs is about 50 but the process can be accelerated by ovarian damage or genetic abnormalities [31].

Follicle Growth

The process of follicle growth can be divided into three stages, each of which has a specific time cycle and specific characteristics. Follicle growth leads to the production of estrogen and the development of a single follicle which will ovulate. Other follicles which do not ovulate become atretic.

First Stage Follicle Growth

This stage is from the primordial follicle with a single layer of flattened pregranulosa cells to the primary follicle which has two or more layers of granulosa cells and a basement membrane separating the granulosa cells from the interstitial tissue of the ovary. First stage growth ends with beginning development of the theca interna. Growth consists of an increase in oocyte size from 15 to 100 μm and an increase in the number of granulosa cells due to mitotic division. The original pregranulosa cells are formed either from germinal epithelium or ovarian stroma, and it is possible that the oocyte produces an organizer substance which induces the formation of granulosa cells. First stage growth does not appear to be related to phases of the ovulation cycle or to other reproductive processes, such as pregnancy or lactation, nor does it appear to be influenced by pituitary gonadotropins, adrenal steroids, or exogenous steroids such as oral contraceptives. As age increases, the rate at which primordial follicles begin first stage growth diminishes. This suggests an intraovarian control mechanism which may somehow be related to the number of follicle units present in the ovary. First stage follicle growth is a self-stimulatory process and goes on continuously from before birth until after menopause.

During first stage follicle growth, five events occur which prepare the follicle for further growth and development: (1) FSH receptors appear in the granulosa cells about the same time the oocyte reaches its maximum size. Once a specific number of receptors per cell has been reached, FSH receptors can be increased only by increasing the number of granulosa cells. (2) Estrogen receptors appear in the granulosa cells at about the same time. Estrogen causes stimulation of granulosa cell mitosis and increases the sensitivity of the granulosa cell adenyl cyclase system to FSH. Adenyl cyclase is involved in the binding of protein hormones to cell membranes. (3) Androgen receptors also appear during first stage follicle development. Little can be said concerning their role except that androgens probably modify the growth and development of the follicle and are involved in the process of atresia. (4) Gap junctions also serve to prepare the follicle for response to external hormone stimuli. These are specialized membrane contacts between granulosa cells and oocyte and among granulosa cells, and it is presumed that they allow exchange of ions and low molecular weight substances among the granulosa cells and between the granulosa cells and the oocyte. (5) At the end of first stage follicle development, when the oocyte has attained a size of about 100 µm and the follicle is about 150–200 µm in diameter, spindle-shaped stromal cells surrounding the follicle become layered outside the basement membrane and develop the histologic characteristic of steroid-secreting cells. The layering effect is probably the result of the expanding follicle and the mechanism which causes the change in histologic appearence is not known. When these histologic changes occur, the cells are known as theca interna cells. As this layer develops, blood vessels and lymphatics proliferate allowing the follicle to be exposed to the hormonal environment of the peripheral plasma. Because of the development of FSH, estrogen and androgen receptors, and the appearance of gap junctions and development of the theca interna, the follicle is now ready to respond to hormonal stimuli [7].

Second Stage Follicle Growth

This stage begins with the development of a fluid-filled cavity called the antrum and ends when the follicle reaches preovulatory size. It occurs during a period of 2–4 weeks and the follicle increases in size from about 200 µm to about 5 mm. The increase in size is from fluid accumulation within the follicle and an increase in the number of granulosa cells. Follicular fluid contains both protein and steroid hormones. Its composition is carefully regulated and probably has an effect on the maturation and development of the follicle and oocyte.

At the end of the luteal phase, as estrogen and progesterone concentrations are decreasing, FSH begins to increase. This serves as a stimulus for a group of several follicles to begin second stage growth. Those follicles which respond are those which have achieved the appropriate degree of development. Soon after ovulation another group of follicles begins to grow, but the rate of growth is considerably slower. Several may reach 3–5 mm in size by the end of the luteal phase, but nearly all will become atretic by the beginning of menses. It is theoretically possible that some follicles, which begin second stage growth after ovulation, may grow very slowly and are ready to respond to increased FSH at the end of the luteal phase. One secondary follicle will reach 5–6 mm about 10–12 days after menses and go into third stage follicle growth and be ovulated. All of the other follicles will become atretic. Thus, the fate of 99.9% of all secondary follicles is to become atretic.

Third Stage Follicle Growth

The beginning of this stage is marked by a spreading apart of the granulosa cells, loosening of the cumulus, and a marked increase in vascularization of the theca interna. It terminates with rupture of the follicle wall and extrusion of the ovum. The follicle increases in size from about 5 to 8–15 mm and the increase is size is due mainly to fluid accumulation. The time period during which third stage growth occurs is 24–48 h. There is no known morphologic difference between the preovulatory follicle and other secondary follicles which will become atretic. There is evidence, however, to indicate that the preovulatory follicle is selected early in the cycle. By the 7th day, blood from the ovarian vein of the ovary which will develop the corpus luteum has a higher concentration of estradiol than ovarian vein blood from the other ovary [2].

Atresia

Atresia is the process of follicle degeneration and is rare in primordial follicles before they begin first stage development. Once the primary follicle stage has been reached, atresia is much more common, and it is the natural fate for all secondary follicles except for one follicle each cycle, which is able to go on to third stage development and be ovulated. The mechanism by which one secondary follicle avoids atresia is unknown although it is probably related to the fact that estrogen tends to prevent atresia and androgen seems to enhance it. It appears that the follicle which is able to maintain a high enough estrogen:androgen ratio is the one which can escape atresia. The site at which atresia begins is not known but probably involves the oocyte in small follicles and the granulosa cells in large follicles. Although the theca cells may degenerate, they commonly show varying degrees of enlargement and even luteinization. It is probable that aggregates of theca cells from atretic follicles form interstitial cells of the ovary.

Hormone Secretion by the Follicle

Any theory of how Graafian follicles grow and secrete estrogen must account for the following facts: (a) both follicle growth and estrogen secretion are exponential; (b) both FSH and LH are required (neither alone is effective); (c) both granulosa and theca cells are required for maximum estrogen secretion; (d) estrogen alone and estrogen plus FSH stimulate

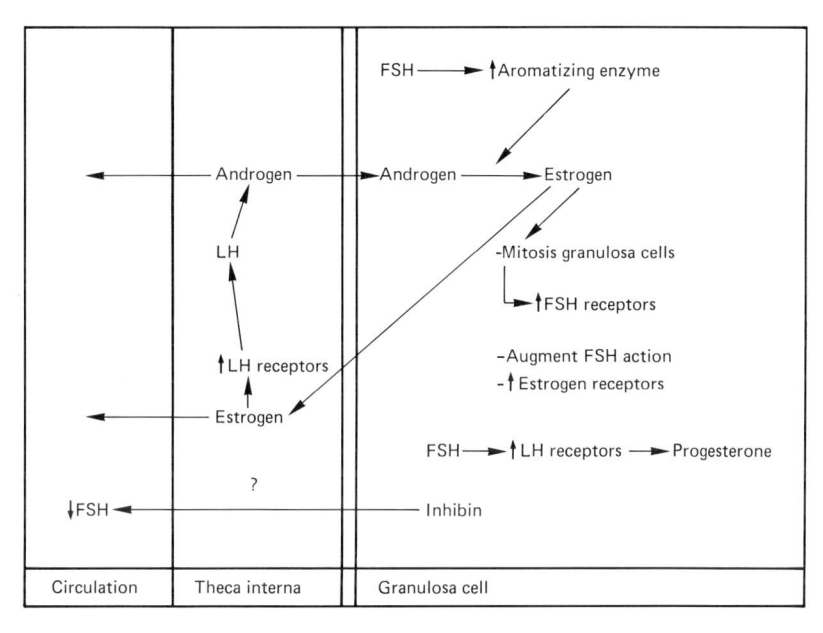

Fig. 2. Two-cell theory of estrogen production by the follicle.

granulosa cell growth; (e) the primary site for LH action is the theca cell, and (f) most of the second stage follicle growth and estrogen secretion can proceed without a change in the rate of secretion of FSH and LH. Until recently, most of these facts were explained by postulating an interaction among FSH, LH, estrogen, granulosa cells, and theca interna. A major part of this theory was that the theca cells were the principal site of estrogen production.

A revised theory is the 'two-cell' theory (fig. 2) which postulates that growth and development of the ovarian follicle involve synergistic interaction between FSH, LH, estrogen, androgen, and granulosa and theca cells and depends in large measure on changes in receptors [18]. As androgen in and around the follicle is converted to estrogen by the aromatase enzyme of the granulosa cell, the increased estrogen produces an increase in estrogen receptors in the granulosa cells and an increase in the number of granulosa cells by stimulating granulosa cell mitosis. Increased numbers of granulosa cells produce an increase in the number of FSH receptors. Estrogen also augments the action of FSH on the granulosa cell by increasing adenyl cyclase which aids in the binding of FSH and other protein hormones. Therefore, a system is established which allows the synergistic action of FSH and estrogen to increase the number of granulosa cells and allow for growth of the follicle and estrogen production.

After exposure to estrogen, FSH receptors increase rapidly because of the growing follicle. Later, FSH causes induction of LH receptors in the granulosa cells and this allows for the production of small amounts of progesterone late in second stage or early third stage growth. The theca interna develops receptors for LH but not FSH, and LH secreted by the pituitary causes the secretion of androstenedione and testosterone from the theca. Androgen diffuses into the granulosa cells where it is converted to estrogen by the aromatase enzyme. Estrogen formed in the granulosa cells diffuse back to the theca and helps to maintain LH receptors. It also gains access to the general circulation via the capillaries which develop in and around the theca cells and basement membrane. As estrogen is produced by the follicle, it tends to stimulate its own production, thereby establishing a self-stimulating mechanism which will produce an exponential rise in estrogen and ultimately stimulate the midcycle LH surge.

The androgen produced in the theca appears to have an inhibitory effect on surrounding follicles and promotes atresia. As estrogen produced by the follicle increases, there is a decrease of FSH because of the inhibitory effect of estrogen on FSH. As FSH decreases, there is a decrease of androgen to estrogen conversion in the granulosa cells. Those follicles which have the most estrogen are the most sensitive to the effects of FSH and better able to maintain androgen to estrogen conversion in the face of decreasing FSH concentrations. The follicle which eventually ovulates is the one which is able to maintain androgen to estrogen conversion at a level which prevents atresia.

The high estrogen tends to augment the actions of FSH. The dominant follicle of the monkey ovary has a better vascularity of the theca than other follicles and this may allow better delivery of FSH to the follicle [39]. This is presumed to be the case in humans also. In fact, most of the estrogen produced during the preovulatory estrogen peak comes from the dominant follicle which will ovulate following the LH surge. The large increase of estrogen over a short period of time triggers the LH surge which is critical to the normal cycle. Failure of the LH surge means failure of ovulation and corpus luteum function and abnormal bleeding or amenorrhea. The LH surge is accompanied by an increase in FSH. The midcycle FSH surge is believed to be due to the small increase of progesterone just before the LH surge (fig. 1) [19, 20] and may be responsible for starting second stage growth of several follicles. The small increase of progesterone is due to the development of LH receptors in the granulosa cells during late second stage follicle development. LH stimulates luteinization of these cells and a shift to progesterone production.

Ovulation and Corpus luteum Formation

Ovulation occurs 20–36 h after the LH surge. The actual process of follicle rupture is poorly understood but seems to involve weakening of the follicle wall. There is evidence in rabbits that contraction of ovarian smooth muscle is involved in the process of ovum extrusion [25, 35]. Intrafollicular prostaglandin may be responsible for this and in the monkey, administration of prostaglandin inhibitors can prevent release of the ovum [11, 24]. A similar mechanism probably exists in the human.

After the LH surge there is a local disintegration in the follicle wall with release of protein enzymes into the extracellular space. The basement membrane of the follicle also begins to degenerate allowing expansion of the preovulatory follicle. This forces the cumulus cells (those granulosa cells which surround the ovum) to separate from the membrana granulosa (those granulosa cells lining the follicle). The ovum and its surrounding cumulus cells become free floating in the follicle and can be extruded. Through a mechanisms not fully understood, the oocyte starts completion of the first meiotic division at the time of the LH surge [4]. This produces a haploid number of chromosomes. Maturation continues to metaphase of the second meiotic division and stops. The process which allows this maturation is probably related to decreased intrafollicular fluid levels of a compound called oocyte maturation-inhibiting factor. After the ovum and its surrounding cumulus has been extruded from the ovary, it should be able to gain entrance into the tube and be transported to the ampullary-isthmic junction where fertilization occurs. The second meiotic division is completed immediately following fertilization and before fusion of the male and female pronuclei. This is also a time of significant hormone change, changes in receptors, and change in the composition of follicular fluid. Although neurotransmitters and releasing hormones are not directly involved in these processes, they are involved in bringing the cycle to the critical stage of ovulation and any chemical or physiologic process which affects the brain may alter the influence of neurotransmitters and releasing factors and disturb the cycle. It should also be remembered that medications not only affect the hypothalamic pituitary relationship but can also be concentrated in follicular fluid and could theoretically affect the ovum and the process of ovulation. If should be noted that the LH surge does not insure ovulation. It it occurs before the follicle is ready to ovulate, luteinization of the granulosa cells may occur without release of an ovum.

Corpus luteum

After ovulation the granulosa cells surrounding the follicle inside the basement membrane become luteinized. This process involves enlargement of the cells and the acquisition of smooth endoplasmic reticulum, mitochondrion with tubovesicular cristae and lipid droplets. The transformation is from small granulosa cells to large cells which have the characteristics of steroid-secreting cells. In the preovulatory follicle, granulosa cells have a poor blood supply because the vascularity of the preovulatory follicle is outside the basement membrane in the theca interna. They are not actively involved in steroid hormone synthesis de novo but are involved in conversion of androgen synthesized in the theca. The luteinized granulosa cells of the corpus luteum are actively involved in synthesis of progesterone and estrogen [9], and are in a well vascularized area.

The corpus luteum secretes large amounts of progesterone which has many effects most or all of which seem to be aimed at supporting pregnancy. Among these effects are changes in cervical mucus and vaginal cytology, an increase of basal body temperature, secretory changes in the endometrium, decreased smooth muscle tone, increased appetite, and increased fatigue. Many of these are experienced to variable degrees by some women as premenstrual changes. In general, progesterone tends to antagonize the effects of estrogen although small amounts of progesterone will frequently augment estrogen activity. In addition to progesterone, the corpus luteum also secretes 17β-estradiol and androstenedione.

The most constant part of the menstrual cycle is the luteal phase – the time from ovulation to the onset of menses. This is because the life span of the corpus luteum is fairly constant at 10–12 days. When corpus luteum function declines and estrogen and progesterone levels diminish, the hormonal basis for endometrial support and maintenance is removed and bleeding ensues. In situations where the length of the cycle varies, that variability is usually in the follicular phase. The corpus luteum is not controlled by another endocrine organ or any known feedback mechanisms and it appears to have its own built-in 'self-destruct' mechanism. The mechanism responsible for corpus luteum regression is not understood. It is thought that prostaglandin F_2 may be involved because it is known to be luteolytic in some mammals [34]. Estrogen also seems to be involved and estrogen injected directly into the ovary causes luteolysis possibly through an effect of prostaglandin on LH receptors [15, 22]. This may be different from spontaneous luteolysis. Normal corpus luteum function does require tonic levels of LH but injections of LH or human chorionic gonadotropin (hCG) will not prolong luteal function indefinitely. However, in normal pregnancy, endogenous hCG will maintain progesterone secretion from the corpus luteum until the placenta is able to supply adequate progesterone at 8 weeks [1, 13].

Control of Gonadotropins

With the discovery of hypothalamic factors which affect the secretion of anterior pituitary hormones, it was assumed that control of the ovulation cycle was in the hypothalamus where complex feedback mechanisms allowed the hypothalamus to control pituitary gonadotropin secretion. Early data in rodents supported the concept that the hypothalamus controlled the pituitary because an increase of GnRH precedes the preovulatory LH surge. It was assumed that the same mechanism exists in humans. The elegant experiments of *Knobil* [16] demonstrated that it was possible to produce a normal ovulatory cycle in monkeys without a midcycle increase of GnRH. The essential factor is that GnRH must be delivered in pulses, the frequency of which is critical. Similar data are not available for humans but there are several bits of indirect evidence which would indicate that the human mechanism is not different from that of the monkey. The concept which has recently emerged is that the real control is in the pituitary. The pituitary needs stimulation from hypothalamic GnRH but the critical factor is the sensitivity of the pituitary to GnRH, which is increased by estrogen, probably through an increase of pituitary GnRH receptors. The pituitary responds to GnRH stimulation by synthesizing and secreting gonadotropins. The degree of pituitary response depends on the ovarian hormones which are produced and secreted in response to pituitary gonadotropic stimulation.

The term 'neurosecretion' refers to the synthesis and release of chemical substances by neurons. Under this definition, nearly all neurons are secretory. Some neurons secrete chemicals such as acetylcholine onto other nerve cells or at the junction of the neuron with glandular or muscle cells. Other neurons may synthesize and release chemicals compounds into the blood. Such substances can be classified as neurohormones by the classic definition of hormones. In the case of the human ovulation cycle, neurohormones are secreted from neurons in the brain in the area of the median eminence. There is a rich capillary network in this area which opens into long portal veins that course down the anterior pituitary. Since there are no direct neuronal connections between the hypothalamus and the anterior pituitary, this hypothalamic-pituitary portal system is the only mechanism for communication between the two organs. This explains how the anterior pituitary gland can be influenced by the nervous system since the anterior pituitary has no secretomotor nerve fibers. The concept is not new. The theory of a hypothalamic pituitary portal chemotransmitter mechanism was discussed over 40 years ago [8, 10] and final proof came with the demonstration that synthetically produced neurohormones had an effect on the secretion of anterior pituitary hormones [12]. The original studies demonstrated that the direction of blood flow in the long portal vessels is from hypothalamus to the pituitary [8]. However, recent studies in rodents [3, 26] indicate that flow may also be retrograde. More specifically it appears that blood flow can be from pituitary to median eminence of the hypothalamus via a network of short portal vessels which drain both anterior and posterior lobes of the pituitary. This would expose the hypothalamus to secretions of both pituitary lobes. Retrograde axonal transport [3, 17] would provide an additional mechanism to expose the hypothalamus to substances in the portal system. The significance of this retrograde portal flow and retrograde axonal transport is not known. It seems reasonable to speculate the presence of feedback mechanisms to the hypothalamus to control the secretion of neurohormones and perhaps modify the effects of neurotransmitters on neurohormone synthesis and release.

Several neurohormones from the hypothalamus have now been identified. Among these are TRH and GnRH. In addition, the median eminence of the hypothalamus contains other biologically active substances including neurotransmitters such as dopamine, norepinephrine, serotonin, acetylcholine, aminobutyric acid, and histamine [29]. GnRH is a decapeptide with a short half-life. Intravenous injection of naturally occurring GnRH or of its synthetic form produces a prompt rise of FSH and LH in humans. The response is proportional to the dose [29] and is influenced by the steroid environment [37, 38]. Endogenous GnRH is synthesized within the hypothalamus by 'peptidergic' cells which respond to neurotransmitters as well as steroid concentrations in the blood. The process is called neurosecretion and involves synthesis of GnRH or other neurohormones or neurotransmitters within the neuron. Synthesis occurs in the endoplasmic reticulum or ribosomes and the substance is packaged into granules in the Golgi apparatus. The granules are transported through the axon and released from nerve endings by reverse pinocytosis [28]. In primates, most of the neurons secreting GnRH have their cell bodies in the medial basal hypothalamus in the area of the arcuate nucleus [33]. GnRH granules travel anteriorly by axonal flow and are secreted into the median eminence at the capillary network of the portal system for transport to the pituitary. Immunocytochemical techniques have identified other tracts of GnRH-secreting fibers descending through the stalk to the posterior pituitary and ascending to the preoptic area. However, it appears that only those GnRh-secreting neurons originating in the arcuate nucleus have an effect on pituitary synthesis and release of gonadotropins.

The basic principles involved in the relationship between the anterior pituitary and the area of the hypothalamus which contains GnRH-secreting neurons was demonstrated in monkeys by *Knobil* [16] and his group. The results of this work indicate that the mechanism in primates is different from that previously observed in rodents. Radiofrequency lesions which destroyed the arcuate nucleus were produced in adult female rhesus monkeys. It had been demonstrated [33] by immunocytochemical techniques that the arcuate nucleus contains the cell bodies of GnRH-secreting neurons. In animals with normal ovarian function given arcuate nucleus lesions, gonadotropin concentrations decreased to unmeasurable levels. Administration of estradiol benzoate did not cause any increase in gonadotropins as noted in animals without arcuate lesions and intact ovaries [36]. In these intact animals, administration of exogenous estrogen produced surges of LH similar to the spontaneous preovulatory LH surges seen in the normal cycle [36].

Continuous infusion of GnRH to ovariectomized animals with an arcuate nucleus lesion produced a transient (12- to 24-hour) increase of FSH and LH which then returned to basal levels if the infusion was continued [27]. If, however, GnRH was given in a pulsatile manner, FSH and LH concentrations remained at preovulatory levels for the duration of the infusion and returned to unmeasurable levels with termination of the infusion. When monkeys with intact ovaries and an arcuate lesion were given a pulsatile infusion of GnRH, the low FSH and LH concentrations caused by the arcuate lesion approached normal, estradiol concentrations began to increase to levels sufficient to cause an LH surge, and subsequent ovulation occurred as indicated by elevated progesterone levels. When ovariectomized animals were studied, there was an increase of gonadotropin following oophorectomy as expected with a drop to unmeasurable levels when the arcuate nucleus lesion was produced. Administration of estradiol did not elicit an LH surge as seen in animals without an arcuate lesion. Once the pulsed GnRH infusion was started in these animals, administration of estradiol benzoate produced a decrease of FSH and LH (inhibitory effect of estrogen) followed by a typical preovulatory surge and return of gonadotropins to lower levels [23].

This suggests that in the monkey, estrogen can exert its negative and positive feedback effects at the level of the pituitary. It also indicates that GnRH must be delivered to the pituitary in pulses in order to have normal pituitary gonadotropin synthesis and release. It is interesting to note that several years ago it was documented that LH release from the pituitary was pulsatile and *Knobil's* group speculated at that time that GnRH release was probably pulsatile [5]. The pulse frequency of GnRH is critical and it appears that once per hour will produce a normal cycle in both monkey and human. It has been demonstrated in monkeys that changing the pulse frequency can alter the concentration of FSH and LH and also have an effect on the FSH:LH ratio. Changing the amplitude of GnRH pulses also changes the concentration of FSH and LH, but the differences are not as dramatic as changing the pulse frequency [16].

Although there is evidence that GnRH does increase in the portal blood in monkeys at the time of the LH surge [16], *Knobil's* work demonstrated that an increase of GnRH at midcycle is not essential. What is important is the concept that pulsed GnRH is necessary to produce normal ovarian follicle growth and subsequent estrogen production. Increasing estrogen increases the pituitary sensitivity to GnRH and allows an LH surge without any change in GnRH synthesis or release. Therefore, control of the menstrual cycle lies in the pituitary and its response to GnRH which is modified by ovarian estrogen secreted as a result of the ovarian response to FSH and LH both of which have to be secreted in a specific pattern.

As noted, there is evidence of an increase of GnRH in the normal cycle and the significance of this is not known. GnRH does have mating effects in male and female animals [29] which may be an important reason for

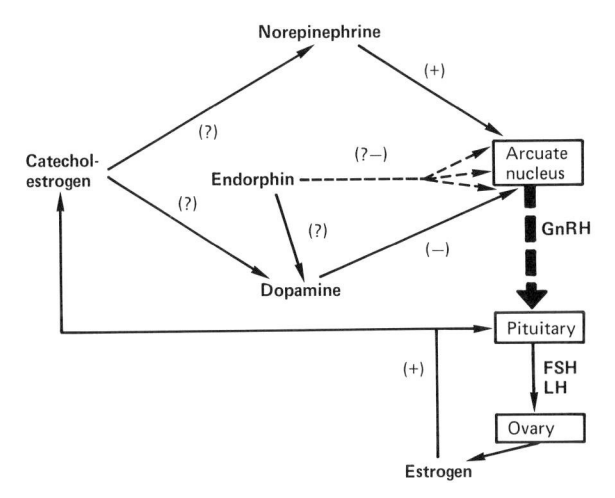

Fig. 3. Summary of hypothalamic-pituitary-ovarian relationship.

elevation of a brain hormone at the time of ovulation. Oophorectomy or estrogen administration in monkeys has no effect on GnRH concentrations in portal blood. The control of GnRH appears to be by other mechanism.

The information derived from monkeys is of vital importance in understanding a very complex mechanism, how it functions and how it may be influenced by pharmacologic and environmental changes. However, the most important question is whether any of this information is applicable to humans. There is circumstantial evidence that the mechanism in humans is similar if not identical to that which has been extensively studied in monkeys and described here (fig. 3).

GnRH is very difficult to measure in humans because the concentration in peripheral blood is so low due to its short half-life. It is not possible of course to obtain samples from the human hypothalamic-pituitary portal circulation. GnRH measured in peripheral blood of humans [6] was noted to have pulsatile increases approximately hourly. The pulses were of much higher magnitude during the periovulatory period that during the follicular or luteal phase of the cycle. Although the authors raise questions about the validity of their methods, the data do fit with what would be expected from our knowledge of the monkey ovulation cycle.

There have been several reports involving the results of the administration of GnRH in humans and its effects on gonadotropin secretion. A report of the administration of GnRH to 2 women with deficient GnRH provides a clinical situation similar to the experimental conditions of *Knobil's* work [30]. GnRH was infused in pulses every 90 min by either the intravenous or subcutaneous route. Intravenous pulses resulted in development of ovarian follicles as measured by ultrasound and in a normal gonadotropin surge with ovulation and subsequent pregnancy. Subcutaneous delivery resulted in abnormal gonadotropin secretion, inadequate follicle development, and no evidence of ovulation. It is possible that higher doses of GnRH given subcutaneously would have produced ovulatory cycles. The important point, however, is that normal ovarian follicle growth and ovulation were produced by pulsatile GnRH administration. This is also compatible with the situation in the monkey. The failure of subcutaneous administration of GnRH to produce normal follicle growth may be because the pituitary did not perceive sharp discrete pulses. More research is obviously needed in this area.

Since it has recently become clear that the ovulation cycle is controlled by the sensitivity of the pituitary to pulsed GnRH and that the pulse frequency, duration, and amplitude of GnRH do not have to change to produce a normal cycle but probably do in the normal physiological situation, it is important to understand the mechanism which controls GnRH secretion. This mechanism is not well understood but there is some information available. The general scheme of fine control of GnRH synthesis and secretion into the portal system involves the catecholamines dopamine and norepinephrine, endogenous opioids, and catecholestrogens.

Anatomic studies have indicated that dopaminergic neurons have cell bodies in the arcuate and paraventricular nuclei with dopamine-secreting neurons ending in the arcuate nucleus and also in the capillary network of the median eminence. It has been shown that intravenous dopamine will decrease both FSH and LH and also prolactin [14]. It appears, therefore, that dopamine may have a direct effect on the GnRH neurons in the arcuate nucleus, probably to change their secretory rate. Through its transport to the pituitary via the portal system, dopamine has a direct effect on the pituitary synthesis and secretion of prolactin. The neurons which secrete norepinephrine terminate in several areas including the hypothalamus where they theoretically could have an effect on the cell bodies of GnRH-secreting neurons or dopaminergic neurons. The current hypothesis is that norepinephrine neurons stimulate GnRH synthesis, and dopamine and serotonin inhibit GnRH. The mechanism probably works by changing the pulse frequency and possibly the amplitude and duration of GnRH secretion. Therefore, any pharmacologic factors which alter catecholamine synthesis or metabolism could theoretically affect the pattern of pulsatile GnRH which reaches the pituitary.

Further modification of the overall system comes from the endogenous opioids which tend to lower gonadotropins and raise prolactin. Endogenous opiates may have an effect on dopmaine neurons and blockade of opiate receptors tends to increase the frequency and amplitude of LH pulses. Although it is not known what happens to GnRH in this situation, it would be reasonable to assume that at least the frequency of GnRH pulses is increased. Endorphins, therefore, appear to modify the interplay between dopamine and norepinephrine. Catecholestrogens provide another modifier for the fine control of this system by interfering with enzymes involved in both synthesis and metabolism of catecholamines. Depending on the enzyme involved, catecholamines could be either decreased or increased. The production of catecholestrogens may be one of the ways steroids modulate the system at the hypothalamic level.

The overall mechanism for the control of GnRH synthesis and secretion is very complex. The primary control seems to be mediated via the catecholamines dopamine and norepinephrine. Although there is no experimental evidence to indicate that GnRH is the result of a balance between dopamine and norepinephrine, the physiologic and anatomic data would be compatible with this concept. Whatever the mechanism, it allows for modification from the environment both emotional and physical, possible feedback by steroids through catecholestrogen and feedback by the hormonal environment of the pituitary via the short portal vessels.

The ovulation cycle in the human functions at several levels and is affected by a variety of factors, both endogenous and exogenous. If the system is working properly, either pregnancy will occur or regular menstrual periods will be present. These are manifestations of ovarian production of estrogen and progesterone in the proper amount and temporal sequence leading to an effect on an end organ such as endometrium, tubal epithelium, vaginal mucosa, pituitary, or any organ which has receptors for these steroids. In order to have appropriate production of estrogen and progesterone it is necessary to have orderly growth and development of ovarian follicles with the emergence of a dominant follicle which releases its ovum. Such normal follicle development depends on stimulation by pituitary gonadotropins in the proper amount and sequence and the interplay between gonadotropins and the estrogen, progesterone and androgen produced by the follicle as it grows. If gonadotropins are not produced in the proper amount and sequence, normal follicle growth and hormone production will not follow. Normal gonadotropin production is dependent on pulsed delivery of GnRH to the pituitary and the sensitivity of the pituitary to GnRH in terms of receptor sites. GnRH secretion in the hypothalamus can be modified by catecholamines, endogenous opiates, catecholestrogens, and a host of physiologic, pharmacologic, and environmental factors. Any abnormality of synthesis, secretion, or receptor binding of releasing hormone, trophic hormone, or sex steroid can affect synthesis, secretion, or binding of the other hormones at other sites and disrupt the delicate balance of a system which is designed to function as an integrated unit and in a self-perpetuating manner. It is not surprising, therefore, that environment, medications, and diseases affect the ovulation cycle and the process of reproduction.

References

1 Atkinson, L.E.; Hotchkiss, J.; Fritz, G.R.; Surue, A.H.; Neill, J.D.; Knobil, E.: Circulating levels of steroids and chorionic gonadotropin during pregnancy in the rhesus monkey, with special attention to the rescue of the corpus luteum in early pregnancy. Biol. Reprod. *12:* 335–345 (1975).
2 Baird, D.T.; Fraser, I.S.: Concentration of oestrone and oestradiol-17β in follicular fluid and ovarian venous blood in women. Clin. Endocrinol. *4:* 259–266 (1975).
3 Bergland, R.M.; Page, R.B.: Can the pituitary secrete directly to the brain? Affirmative anatomic evidence. Endocrinology *102:* 1325–1338 (1978).
4 Channing, C.P.; Schaerf, F.W.; Anderson, L.D.; Tsafriri, A.: Ovarian follicular and luteal physiology. Int. Rev. Physiol. *22:* 117–201 (1980).
5 Dierschke, D.J.; Bhattacharya, A.N.; Atkinson, L.E.; Knobil, E.: Circhoral oscillations of plasma LH levels in the ovariectomized rhesus monkey. Endocrinology *87:* 850–853 (1970).
6 Elkind-Hirsch, K.; Ravhikar, V.; Schiff, I.; Tulchinsky, D.; Ryan, K.J.: Determinations of endogenous immunoreactive luteinizing hormone-releasing hormone in human plasma. J. clin. Endocr. Metab. *54:* 602–607 (1982).
7 Erickson, G.F.: Normal ovarian function. Clin. Obstet. Gynec. *21:* 31–52 (1978).
8 Fink, G.: The development of the releasing factor concept. Clin. Endocrinol. *5:* suppl., pp. 245s–260s (1976).
9 Fritz, M.A.; Speroff, L.: Current concepts of the endocrine characteristics of normal menstrual function: the key to diagnosis and management of menstrual disorders. Clin. Obstet. Gynec. *26:* 647–689 (1983).
10 Green, J.D.; Harris, G.W.: Neurovascular link between neurohypophysis and adenohypophysis. J. Endocr. *5:* 136–146 (1947).
11 Grenwich, D.L.; Kennedy, T.G.; Armstrong, D.T.: Dissociation of ovulatory and steroidogenic actions of luteinizing hormone in rabbits with indomethacin: an inhibitor of prostaglandin biosynthesis. Prostaglandins *1:* 89–96 (1972).

12 Guillemin, R.: Peptides in the brain: the new endocrinology of the neuron. Science *202:* 390–402 (1978).
13 Jaffe, R.B.; Lee, P.A.; Midgley, A.R.: Serum gonadotropins before, at the inception of, and following human pregnancy. J. clin. Endocr. Metab. *29:* 1281–1284 (1969).
14 Judd, S.J.; Rakoff, J.S.; Yen, S.S.C.: Inhibition of gonadotropin and prolactin release by dopamine: effect of endogenous estradiol levels. J. clin. Endocr. Metab. *47:* 494–498 (1978).
15 Karsch, F.J.; Sutton, G.P.: An intraovarian site for the luteolytic action of estrogen in the rhesus monkey. Endocrinology *98:* 553–561 (1976).
16 Knobil, E.: The neuroendocrine control of the menstrual cycle. Recent Prog. Horm. Res. *36:* 53–88 (1980).
17 LaVail, J.H.; LaVail, M.M.: Retrograde axonal transport in the central nervous system. Science *176:* 1416–1417 (1972).
18 Makris, A.; Ryan, K.J.: Progesterone, androstenedione, testosterone, estrone and estradiol synthesis in hamster ovarian follicle cells. Endocrinology *96:* 694–701 (1975).
19 March, C.M.; Goebelsmann, U.; Nakamura, R.M.; Mishell, D.R.: Roles of estradiol and progesterone in eliciting the midcycle luteinizing hormone and follicle stimulating hormone surges. J. clin. Endocr. Metab. *49:* 507–513 (1979).
20 March, C.M.; Marrs, R.P.; Goebelsmann, U.; Mishell, D.R.: Feedback effects of estradiol and progesterone upon gonadotropin and prolactin release. Obstet. Gynec., N.Y. *58:* 10–16 (1981).
21 McCann, S.M.; Dhariwal, A.P.S.: Hypothalamic releasing factors and the neurovascular link between the brain and the anterior pituitary; in Martini, Ganong, Neuroendocrinology, vol. 1, pp. 261–296 (Academic Press, New York 1966).
22 Najano, R.; Yamoto, M.; Iwasaki, M.: Effects of oestrogen and prostaglandin $F_{2\alpha}$ on luteinizing hormone receptors in human copora lutea. J. Endocr. *88:* 401–408 (1981).
23 Nakai, Y.; Plant, T.M.; Hess, D.L.; Keogh, E.J.; Knobil, E.: On the sites of the negative and positive feedback actions of estradiol in the control of gonadotropin secretion in the rhesus monkey. Endocrinology *102:* 1008–1014 (1978).
24 O'Grady, J.P.; Caldwell, B.V.; Auletta, F.J.; Speroff, L.: The effects of an inhibitor of prostaglandin synthesis (indomethacin) on ovulation, pregnancy and pseudopregnancy in the rabbit. Prostaglandins *1:* 97–106 (1972).
25 Okamura, H.; Virutamasen, P.; Wright, H.; Wallach, E.E.: Ovarian smooth muscles in the human being, rabbit and cat. Histochemical and electron microscopic study. Am. J. Obstet. Gynec. *112:* 183–191 (1972).
26 Oliver, C.; Mical, R.S.; Porter, J.C.: Hypothalamic pituitary vasculature: evidence for retrograde flow in the pituitary stalk. Endocrinology *101:* 589–604 (1977).
27 Plant, T.M.; Krey, L.C.; Moossy, J,; McCormick, J.T.; Hess, D.L.; Knobil, E.: The arcuate nucleus and the control of gonadotropins and prolactin secretion in the female rhesus monkey *(Macaca mulatta)*. Endocrinology *102:* 52–62 (1978).
28 Reichlin, S.: Neuroendocrinology; in Williams, Textbook of endocrinology; 6th ed., pp. 589–645 (Saunders, Philadelphia 1981).
29 Reichlin, S.: Neuroendocrinology of pituitary regulation; in Givens, Hormone-secreting pituitary tumors, pp. 1–26 (Yearbook Medical Publishers, Chicago 1982).
30 Reid, R.L.; Leopold, G.R.; Yen, S.S.C.: Induction of ovulation and pregnancy with pulsatile luteinizing hormone releasing factor: dosage and mode of delivery. Fert. Steril. *36:* 553–559 (1981).

31 Ross, G.T.; Vande Wiele, R.L.; Frantz, A.G.: The ovaries and the breasts; in Williams, Textbook of endocrinology; pp. 355–360 (Saunders, Philadelphia 1981).
32 Schally, A.V.: Aspects of hypothalamic regulation of the pituitary gland: its implications for the control of reproductive processes. Science *202:* 18–28 (1978).
33 Silverman, A.J.; Antunes, J.L.; Ferin, M.; Zimmerman, E.A.: The distribution of LHRH in the hypothalamus of the rhesus monkey. Light microscopic studies using immunoperoxidase technique. Endocrinology *101:* 134–142 (1977).
34 Sotrel, G.; Helvacioglu, A.L.; Dowers, S.; Scommegna, A.; Auletta, F.J.: Mechanism of luteolysis: effect of estradiol and prostaglandin $F_{2\alpha}$ on corpus luteum luteinizing hormone-human chorionic gonadotropin receptors and cyclic nucleotides in the rhesus monkey. Am. J. Obstet. Gynec. *139:* 134–140 (1981).
35 Virutamasen, P.; Wright. K.H.; Wallach, E.E.: Effects of prostaglandin E_2 and $F_{2\alpha}$ on ovarian contractility in the rabbit. Fert. Steril. *23:* 675–682 (1972).
36 Yamaji, T.; Dierschke, D.J.; Hotchkiss, J.; Bhattachanya, A.H.; Sarve, A.H.; Knobil, E.: Estrogen induction of LH release in the rhesus monkey. Endocrinology *89:* 1034–1041 (1971).
37 Yen, S.S.C.; Vandenberg, G.; Silver, T.M.: Modulation of pituitary responsiveness to LRF by estrogen. J. clin. Endocr. Metab. *39:* 170–177 (1974).
38 Young, J.R.; Jaffe, R.B.: Strength duration characteristics of estrogen effects on gonadotropin response to gonadotropin-releasing hormone in women. II. Effects of varying concentrations of estradiol. J. clin. Endocr. Metab. *43:* 432–442 (1976).
39 Zeleznik, A.J.; Schuler, H.M.; Reichert, L.E.: Gonadotropin binding sites in the rhesus monkey ovary: role of the vasculature in the selective distribution of human chorionic gonadotropin to the preovulatory follicle. Endocrinology *109:* 356–362 (1981).

Paul T. Schnatz, MD, Department of Reproductive Biology, Case Western Reserve University School of Medicine, Head, Division of Reproductive Endocrinology and Infertility, University Hospitals, Cleveland, OH 44106 (USA)

Psychoendocrinology and the Menstrual Cycle

David D. Youngs[a, b], *Nancy Reame*[c]

[a] Departments of Obstetrics/Gynecology and Psychiatry, Maine Medical Center, Portland, Me.; [b] Department of Obstetrics and Gynecology, University of Vermont, Burlington, Vt.; [c] Department of Internal Medicine, University of Michigan, Ann Arbor, Mich., USA

Sociocultural Perspectives

Menstruation in contrast to many important bodily functions is commonly invested with a variety of sociocultural, ethnic, and other highly personal beliefs [21]. Depending upon such beliefs, what constitutes normal vs. abnormal menstruation may be perceived quite differently by individual patients and physicians. As has been so poignantly expressed in literature, a women's menses represent a very personal experience colored by both negative and positive emotions. Important insights into the variety of experiences women associate with menstruation have been reported by *Abplanalp* [1], *Chernovetz* et al. [6] and *Whisnant* et al. [36]. These authors and others have drawn attention to the importance of the mother/daughter relationship and particular sociocultural influences in shaping an adolescent's view about menstrual function.

Although scientific data are lacking, anecdotal reports suggest that some women can deliberately extend their menstrual cycle length, that others participating regularly in team sports may synchronize their menstrual cycles to within a few days of each other, and that family members vacationing together may establish a common menstrual cycle.

With the growing interest of women in both competitive and noncompetitive sports, of more practical concern to the practicing gynecologist are exercise-associated menstrual alterations [27, 32]. *Frisch and Revel* [11] propose that body weight, particularly lean body mass, is of critical importance, both in the initiation and maintenance of menstrual function. The *Frisch* 'critical weight hypothesis' has been proposed as an explanation for the amenorrhea commonly seen with competitive physical and athletic activities, as in gymnasts, ballet dancers, marathon runners, as well as young women with anorexia nervosa. However, the studies by *Shangold* [30] and *Schwartz* et al. [27] on female distance and marathon runners indicate that oligo- and amenorrhea often exist even before competitive running begins. Further, *Katz and Weiner* [16] in their work on anorexia nervosa report amenorrhea before weight loss occurs, and also that return to normal weight was not necessarily associated with resumption of menstruation. *Warren* [34], in her studies on adolescent ballet dancers, found prepubertal changes, particularly menarche and secondary sex changes, markedly delayed during active training. Initiation of menstruation and progression of sexual development begin in two-thirds (10/15) of her sample only with a decrease in exercise or forced rest from an injury of at least 2 months duration. Interestingly, during the interval that menstruation began, changes in body weight and lean body mass were minimal or absent. Although an attractive explanation, the *Frisch* hypothesis appears insufficient to account for many of the observations made on exercise-associated menstrual dysfunctions.

Weiner et al. [35] in their investigations into psychosomatic mechanisms of disease, suggest that 'health is associated with certain patterns of sleep, hormone and neurotransmitter release...'. They go on to point out that 'it is only recently recognized that some diseases may be associated with shifts in phase, or ... age-inappropriate patterns of these rhythmic physiologic functions. This way of viewing disease goes beyond the usual manner of looking for an anatomical lesion or some quantitative alteration, such as the absence of or structural alteration of an enzyme as a full explanation of pathological anatomy or pathophysiology of disease'. It is within this broader psychosomatic framework that this paper will focus.

Psychosomatic Concepts Relevant to the Management of Menstrual Dysfunction

An understanding of psychosomatic concepts may be useful to the gynecologist when evaluating patients with complaints for which underlying organic factors are not readily apparent, or are insufficient to explain the patient's level of distress. Not uncommonly, such complaints are diagnosed as functional or 'psychosomatic' without further exploration. Rarely are patients satisfied with this approach, and therapeutic efforts frequently fail. For example, in an individual for which initial investigation has failed to reveal an underlying cause of excessive menstrual bleeding, a clinician may wish to alter his line of inquiry and ask the following questions. (1) What are the patient's concerns about the particular presenting complaint? What is her explanation about what may be wrong? For example, is she afraid that abnormal bleeding may suggest an underlying cancer or recent injury from intercourse? Is there guilt about sexual behavior? (2) Are there socioenvironmental stress factors, operative in the patient's daily life, which may be contributing to the presenting complaint? (3) What purpose might the symptoms serve in this particular patient? For example avoiding work, family responsibilities, or intercourse. (4) Is there reason to consider a more biologic presentation when current lifestyle does not suggest significant underlying emotional turmoil?

In such circumstances, a variety of psychosocial dynamics may be present, the more common of which relate to concerns about sexual or reproductive function, interpersonal relationships, and/or career-occupational conflicts. With the above information in hand, the physician can better determine the need for a more concentrated exploration of the patient's daily life experiences and socioenvironmental setting, or further diagnostic or surgical intervention.

For many physicians, working in the psychosomatic mode can be distressing, particularly for those who wish to establish a prompt diagnosis and initiate specific therapy. When faced with a difficult and confusing diagnostic problem, one might ask, how does the patient make the physician feel? Certainly personal reactions of frustration, anger, or a sense of not being able to satisfy the patient, should alert the clinician to potential problems in the doctor/patient relationship. Either such patients trigger an idiosyncratic reaction in the physician or may reflect the presence of underlying emotional or social/situational factors. As we have noted, working with such patients involves a cognitive switch from being an objective diagnostician to standing back, getting a feeling for the patient, and what meaning such symptoms may have in her particular circumstances.

In brief, psychosomatic medicine does not focus exclusively on questions for 'cause and effect' but rather places patients and their health problems within a broader social and behavioral context. And finally, it bears emphasizing that psychosomatic facets exist in most, if not all diseases [35].

A Theoretical Framework for Psychosomatic Medicine

Near the turn of the century, *Virchow* [38] observed that knowledge of chemistry would become indispensable to the practice of medicine, however, at the time chemistry had nothing of practical value to offer. The evolution of psychosomatic concepts in medicine has follow a similar history. *Selye* [29], in the late 1930s, experimentally demonstrated that the response of the body to stress depends on the brain. More recently, *Mason* has established a relationship between environmental stress and subtle, rapid, and specific fluctuations in various endocrine functions. Other more contemporary investigators including *Stein* et al. [33], *Wolf*, and *Weiner* et al. [35] have further documented the importance of brain mechanisms in the control of the autonomic nervous system, neuroendocrine activity, and both humoral and cell-mediated immunological responses. Research in psychosomatic medicine has shifted from a preoccupation with specificity hypotheses (i.e. that a particular personality type may be associated with a specific physical disease), psychoanalytic explanations of illness, and the use of psychoanalysis on patients with organic disease. Increasingly research in this area has come to focus on environmental stresses, a broader variety of physical diseases, and specific disease mechanisms.

Psychosomatic Reproductive Endocrinology

Brain-Body Interrelationships
Theoretically, brain mechanisms can alter menstruation and reproductive function through a variety of pathways, including neuroendocrine, autonomic, immunologic, or other biochemical mediators. Preliminary data suggest that several of the above mechanisms may be of etiologic importance in psychosomatic aspects of menstrual dysfunction. Since *Schildkraut,* in 1965, first hypothesized that brain neurotransmitters (biogenic amines) are of etiologic importance in certain psychiatric disorders, particularly depression, psychiatrists and neurobiologists have become increasingly interested in an area of the brain commonly referred to as the limbic system. While not identified as a specific division of the brain, the limbic system appears to represent a locus of neurochemical and neurophysiological activity that is both functionally and anatomically related. Basic human survival behaviors including the response to a

perceived threat, eating and sleeping, as well as sexual and reproductive functions appear to be intimately relative to limbic system activity.

In brief, the limbic system is perceived by many psychiatrists as the 'emotional brain', an area found to be of increasing importance in linking higher cortical functions with autonomic, neuroendocrine, and other involuntary responses. While psychosomatic mechanisms have been most thoroughly investigated in a select number of diseases including hypertension, asthma, peptic disease, and anorexia nervosa, disorders of the female reproductive system have increasingly come under scrutiny.

It has been well documented that emotional stress can disrupt ovarian function and induce infertility. Stress has been cited as the cause of disturbances in the timing of ovulation during the month that artificial insemination was anticipated [10]. As reviewed by *Drew* [9], there appears to be a high incidence of secondary amenorrhea under stress environmental conditions, such as among factory workers, Air Force and Navy recruits, and hospitalized patients with psychiatric illness. Although the duration of posttraumatic amenorrhea following high level spinal cord injury may extend for up to several years, a large percentage of quadriplegic women experience no interruption of menses, suggesting that socioenvironmental stress may significantly influence the timing of menstrual cycle return [7].

Psychogenic amenorrhea has been associated with a variety of abnormal gonadotropin patterns and estrogen-deficient symptoms suggesting polycystic ovarian disease or premature menopause. Sociopsychologic distress may play a role in the elevation of prolactin secretion and acyclic gonadotropin patterns seen in women with post-pill galactorrhea-amenorrhea; when psychologic dysfunction was corrected through psychiatric counseling, normal hormonal function resumed [40]. In pseudocyesis, a condition characterized by prolactin hypersecretion, a similar mechanism may be operative [20].

Brain Catecholamines

Psychogenic-induced menstrual cycle disorders may result from disruption of the neuroendocrine integrating system that controls reproduction, referred to as the hypothalamo-pituitary-ovarian axis. At the level of the hypothalamus, it is believed that gonadotropin-releasing hormone (GnRH) is regulated by a dual catecholaminergic system in which dopamine (DA) exerts inhibitory effects and norepinephrine (NE) exerts facilitatory effects on GnRH release. In addition, these two neurotransmitters appear to undergo cyclic changes in central activity coincident with the midcycle LH surge [39].

There is growing evidence to suggest that situational or emotional distress may promote or enhance an imbalance in brain biogenic amine formations and metabolism. Experiments in laboratory animals using a variety of stress-inducing techniques have shown that both acute and chronic stress can enhance brain catecholamine formation through stimulation of the rate-limiting first step in production involving tyrosine hydroxylase (TOH). One of the ways this effect may be mediated is through the action of stress-induced secretion of adrenal glucocorticoids which have been shown to influence the steady-state levels of brain TOH [4]. Stress in animals has also been shown to produce a decrease in monoamine oxidase activity in the hypothalamus, thus prolonging the action of brain catecholamines [23].

Dopaminergic hyperfunction in the hypothalamus could result in inhibition of GnRH release and suppression of ovulation. In humans, administration of DA or DA agonists such as *L*-dopa and bromocriptine produce a dramatic suppression of the midcycle LH surge [39]. Women diagnosed with low-weight amenorrhea and who received the dopamine receptor antagonist metaclopramide showed a significantly elevated LH response to GnRH stimulation, suggesting increased central dopaminergic activity in this condition [18].

There is growing evidence to suggest that another biogenic amine found in high concentrations in the hypothalamus may play a role in stress-mediated events. Secretion of the endogenous amine β-phenethylamine (PEA), which resembles amphetamine both structurally and pharmacologically, has been shown to be markedly elevated in schizophrenic patients as well as in normal males and females in response to parachute jumping [22, 24]. A relationship between stress-induced PEA secretion and menstrual dysfunction in women remains to be investigated.

Endogenous Opiates

A number of endogenous compounds in the brain have been purported to act as modulators of central neurotransmitter function to amplify, dampen, or set the tone of local synaptic activity by altering the effectiveness of a neurotransmitter [4]. The endogenous opiate peptides may play a role in stress-induced dysfunction. Studies in normal women as well as those with hypothalamic amenorrhea suggest that β-endorphin suppresses LH while augmenting prolactin secretion [20]. *Blankstein* et al. [5] postulate that excessive endorphin secretion may be involved in the pathophysiology of secondary amenorrhea and hyperprolactinemia, since naloxone administration to women with these conditions elicited a significant increase in serum LH. No response was elicited in women with GnRH deficiency, suggesting that naloxone acts normally by uncovering the inhibitory action of an endogenous opioids pathway upon hypothalamic GnRH secretion. Opioids may increase pituitary prolactin through their inhibitory interaction with dopamine nerve terminals in the median eminence [15, 28]. A single large precursor molecular 'proopiocortin' appears to be the prohormone for ACTH, α-MSH (melanocyte-stimulating hormone), β-LPH, and β-endorphin [17]. A current hypothesis that is supported by animal and human studies suggests that β-endorphin is released simultaneously with ACTH from the pituitary in response to stress. This ACTH-linked release is believed to provide stress-induced analgesia to dampen the perception of pain during threatening circumstances [19, 37]. In the rat, the maternal pain threshold has been shown to rise progressively during pregnancy and can be suppressed by the administration of a narcotic antagonist. No changes were observed in nonpregnant animals, suggesting a pregnancy-specific response that is mediated by an endorphin system [13]. In nonpregnant women, plasma concentrations of β-endorphin are not significantly different from male values; during pregnancy they rise progressively, reaching maximal values at delivery. The placenta has been implicated as the secretory source of this pregnancy-specific phenomenon [12].

β-Endorphin may also act as a neuromodulator of the well-known stress-associated increase in vasopressin (VP) secretion. *Reid and Yen* [26] cite animal and human evidence for a stimulatory effect of endogenous opiates on vasopressin secretion which they implicate as a major causative agent in the physical and emotional symptoms of the premenstrual distress syndrome. Women with dysmenorrhea demonstrate a significantly higher plasma concentration of VP on day 1 of the cycle than do asymptomatic controls [2].

Prolactin

A significant relationship exists between emotional stress and hyperprolactinemia [28]. Some researchers argue that this stress-related reflex is mediated through hypothalamic serotonergic neurons which increase prolactin-releasing factor secretion. Increased prolactin levels have been shown to suppress gonadotropin cyclicity and induce anovulation and amenorrhea probably as a result of local as well as central inhibition of the reproductive cycle [8]. In contrast, the hyperprolactinemia and elevated gonadotropin secretion are associated with pseudocyesis is believed to result from a deficiency of hypothalamic dopaminergic activity since the administration of dopa agonists can suppress hypersecretion [39]. Hyperprolactinemia has also been associated with luteal phase shortening as a result of a direct effect on ovarian progesterone production [3]. This mechanism could account for the commonly observed 'honeymoon' phenomenon of stress-induced menses onset.

Other endogenous compounds that have been implicated as possible neuromodulators of stress-mediated menstrual dysfunction include melatonin from the pineal gland, MSH from the intermediate lobe of the pituitary, testosterone [30], and hypothalamic catechol estrogens [8, 26].

In summary, it appears that there exists a variety of mechanisms whereby psychosomatic factors can lead to alterations in central neurotransmitters and/or neuroregulators of the reproductive axis resulting in menstrual and reproductive cycle dysfunction.

Conclusions

Patients reporting disturbances of menstruation continue to make up a significant proportion of gynecologic practice. In the not too distant past, menstrual disorders were managed by either empiric medical or surgical therapies, with little understanding of specific etiologic factors. Contemporary knowledge of gynecologic endocrinology and pathology have significantly extended the clinicians' understanding and choices of therapy for menstrual complaints.

Unfortunately, a number of patients continue to present with problems of menstruation for which no apparent organic abnormality can be found, while others appear to demonstrate a clear-cut menstrual disorder but fail to respond to accepted therapy. An additional group of patients present with a confusing clinical picture with contradictory historical, physical, or laboratory findings. In just such situations, a psychosomatic perspective is proposed. Important life eyperiences, socioenvironmental stresses, and emotional factors may be productively explored within a psychobiological context.

Recognition is given to the fact that diseases are often heterogeneous and multifactorial in nature; further, that brain mechanisms most likely play a role in some stage of most diseases, particularly disturbances of the reproductive and menstrual cycle; and finally, that psychosomatic principes of diagnosis and management are not to be confused with intuitive or common sense approaches, but increasingly rest on a well-established foundation of behavioral science research.

References

1 Abplanalp, J.: The menstrual cycle: costs and Benefits. 10th Annu. Conf. Psychosom. Obstet. Gynec., San Francisco 1982.
2 Akerlund, J.; Stromberg, P.; Forsling, M.L.: Primary dysmenorrhea and vasopressin. Br. J. Obstet. Gynaec. *86:* 484 (1979).
3 Balmaceda, M.P.; Eddy, C.A.; Smith, C.G.; Asch, R.H.: The effects of hyperprolactinemia on the luteal phase of the rhesus monkey. Endocrine and Fertility Forum, vol. V (Feb.), 1982. Rep. 29th, Annu. Meet. Pacific Coast Fertil. Soc. (1982).
4 Barchas, J.D.; Akil, H.; Elliot, G.R.; Holman, R.B.; Watson, S.J.: Behavioral neurochemistry: neuroregulators and behavioral states. Science *200:* 964 (1978).
5 Blankstein, J.; Reyes, F.I.; Winter, J.S.D.; Faiman, C.: Endorphins and the regulation of the human menstrual cycle. Clin. Endocrinol. *14:* 287 (1981).
6 Chernovetz, M.E.; Jones, W.H.; Hanson, R.O.: Predictability, attentional focus, sex role orientation, and menstrual-related stress. Psychosom. Med. *41:* 383 (1979).
7 Comarr, A.E.P.: Interesting observations of females with spinal cord injury. Med. Servs J. Can. *22:* 651 (1966).
8 Cutler, W.B.; Garcia, C.R.: The pychoneuroendocrinology of the ovulatory cycle of women: a review. Psychoneuroendocrines *5:* 89 (1980).
9 Drew, F.L.: The epidemiology of secondary amenorrhea. J. Chron. Dis. *14:* 396 (1961).
10 Foldes, J.J.: Ovulatory disturbances of psychosomatic origin., in: The family, 4th Int. Congr. Psychosom. Obstet. Gynec., pp. 330–333 (Karger, Basel 1975).
11 Frisch, R.E.; Revel, E.R.: Height and weight at menarche and a hypothesis of critical body weights and adolescent events. Science *169:* 397 (1970).
12 Gennazani, A.R.; Facchinetti, F.; Parrini, D.: Beta-lipotrophin and beta-endorphin plasma levels during pregnancy. Clin. Endocrinol. *14:* 409 (1981).
13 Gintzler, A.R.: Endorphin-mediated increase in pain threshold during pregnancy. Science *210:* 193 (1980).
14 Groll, M.: Gonadotropic patterns in psychogenic amenorrhea. Int. J. Gyneac. Obstet. *16:* 53 (1978).
15 Iwamoto, E.T.; Way, E.L.: Opiate actions and catecholamines. Biochem. Psychol. *20:* 357 (1979).
16 Katz, J.L.; Weiner, H.: The aberrant reproductive endocrinology of anorexia nervosa; in Weiner, Hofer, Stundark, Brain, behavior and bodily disease (Raven Press, New York 1981).
17 Krieger, D.T.; Liotta, A.S.: Pituitary hormones in the brain: where, how and why? Science *205:* 366 (1979).
18 Larsen, S.: Responses of luteinizing hormone, follicle stimulating hormone, and prolactin to prolonged administration of a dopamine antagonist in normal women and women with low-weight amenorrhea, Fert. Steril. *35:* 642 (1981).
19 Marx, J.L.: Analgesia: how the body inhibits pain perception. Science *195:* 741 (1977).
20 McFalls, J.A.: Psychopathology and subfecundity (Academic Press, New York 1979).
21 Parlee, J.: Social and emotional aspects of menstruation, birth and menopause; in Youngs, Ehrhardt, Psychosomatic Obstetrics and Gynecology (Appleton Century Croft, New York 1980).

22   Paulos, M.A.; Tessel, R.E.: Excretion of beta phenethylamine is elevated in humans after profound stress. Science *215:* 1127 (1982).
23   Petrovic, V.M.; Sibalic, V.J.: in Usdin et al., Catecholamines and stress: recent advances, p 365. (Elsevier, New York 1980).
24   Potkin, S.G.; Karoum, F.; Chuang, L.W.; Cannon-Spoor, H.E.; Phillips, I.L.; Wyatt, R.J.: Phenethylamine in paranoid chronic schizophrenia. Science *206:* 470 (1979).
25   Quigley, M.E.; Sheehan, K.L.; Casper, R.F.; Yen, S.S.C.: Evidence for increased dopaminergic and opioid activity in patients with hypothalamic hypogonadotropic amenorrhea. J. clin. Endocr. Metab. *50:* 949 (1980).
26   Reid, R.L.; Yen, S.S.C.: Premenstrual syndrome. Am. J. Obstet. Gynec. *139:* 85 (1981).
27   Schwartz, B.; Cumming, D.C.; Riordan, E.; Seiye, M.; Yen, S.C.; Rebar, R.W.: Exercise associated amenorrhea. A distinct entity? Am. J. Obstet. Gynec. *141:* 662 (1981).
28   Seibel, M.M.; Taymor, M.L.: Emotional aspects of infertility. Fert. Steril. *37:* 137 (1982).
29   Selye, H.: The stress of life: a new theory of disease (McGraw-Hill, New York 1956).
30   Shangold, M.: The effect of marathon training upon menstrual function, Am. J. Obstet. Gynec. (accepted for publication).
31   Singh, D.B.: Menstrual disorders in college students. Am. J. Obstet. Gynec. *140:* 299 (1981).
32   Speroff, L.; Redwine, D.B.: Exercise and menstrual function, Physician Sportsmed. *8:* 42 (1980).
33   Stein, M.; Schiavi, R.C.; Camerino, M.S.: Influence of brain and behavior on the immune system. Science *191:* 435 (1976).
34   Warren, M.P.: The effects of exercise on pubertal progress and reproductive functions in girls. J. clin. Endocr. Metab. *41:* 1150 (1980).
35   Weiner, H.; Hofer, M.S.; Stunkard, A.J.: Brain, behavior and bodily disease (Raven Press, New York 1981).
36   Whisnant, L.; Breet, E.; Zagans, L.: Implicit messages concerning menstruation in commercial educational materials prepared for young adolescent girls. Am. J. Psychiat. *132:* 815 (1975).
37   Wiler, J.C.; Dehen, H.; Cambier, J.: Stress-induced analgesia in humans: endogenous opioids and naloxone reversible depression of pain reflexes. Science *232:* 689 (1981).
38   Virchow, R.: Disease, life and man; transl. Rathers, L.J. (Stanford University Press, Stanford 1958).
39   Yen, S.S.C.: Neuroendocrine regulation of the menstrual cycle. Hosp. Pract. *14:* 83 (1979).
40   Zacur, H.A.; Chapanis, N.P.; Lake, C.R.; Ziegler, M.; Tyson, J.E.: Galactrorrhea-amenorrhea: psychological interaction with neuroendocrine function. Am. J. Obstet. Gynec. *125:* 859 (1976).

David D. Youngs, MD, Maine Medical Center, Portland, ME (USA)

Pathophysiologic Basis for the Menopause

John DeFazio[a, b], Cynthia Austin[a, c], Leon Speroff[d, e]

[a] Department of Obstetrics and Gynecology, Case Western Reserve University School of Medicine; [b] Division of Reproductive Endocrinology and Infertility, University Hospitals of Cleveland, Ohio; [c] Division of Endocrinology and Fertility; [d] Department of Reproductive Biology, Case Western Reserve University School of Medicine; [e] Department of Obstetrics and Gynecology, University Hospitals of Cleveland, Ohio, USA

Profound changes in reproductive function are associated with aging in women. The most traumatic is cessation of ovarian follicular maturation. This event, the menopause, is marked by the discontinuation of menstruation and is associated with a constellation of endocrinologic, physiologic, and psychologic symptoms. Many of these are specifically relieved by estrogen replacement therapy. This chapter addresses the pathophysiologic basis for these symptoms and the potential benefits and risks of estrogen and alternative nonestrogen therapies.

According to the Bureau of Census' figures for 1979, there were 32 million women over the age of 50 in the United States. Because the average age of menopause in women is 51 years, most of these women have had or shortly will have their last menstrual cycle. Statistics indicate that the life expectancy of women in the United States is 81 years. Younger women also can have ovarian failure because of spontaneous cessation or surgical removal. Thus, many women do not have ovarian function and live about one-third of their lives after menopause.

Mechanisms of Menopause

In the female, oogenesis begins in the fetal ovary at approximately the 3rd week of gestation [1]. At 20 weeks gestation, the fetal ovaries contain approximately 7 million oogonia [2]. After 7 months of gestation no new oocytes are formed. From then until the menopause, the number of germ cells falls steadily. At birth there are approximately 2 million oocytes, and by puberty this number has been reduced to 300,000. Two processes, ovulation and atresia, are responsible for the continued reduction of oocyte number during the reproductive years. Atresia accounts for the loss of 90% of oocytes whereas only 400 oocytes are ovulated. Very little is known about oocyte atresia.

Menopause occurs in human females because follicles that are responsive to gonadotropins are no longer present. Remaining follicles do not respond to gonadotropins. Isolated occytes can be found in postmenopausal ovaries by careful histological examination [3]. Few of the remaining follicles show development and the majority are atretic.

Endocrinologic Changes of the Menopause

Estrogens

After the menopause, there is obvious clinical evidence of reduced estrogen production in most women. When circulating levels of estrogen have been assessed, the greatest decrease has been found in estradiol. Most investigators find a mean concentration of approximately 13 pg/ml [4–6]. This level is similar to that seen in premenopausal women following oophorectomy [7, 8]. The source of the small amount of estradiol found in menopausal women has not been well established. Direct secretion by the ovary does not appear to contribute significantly since circulating levels are similar before and after oophorectomy [7, 8]. The adrenal glands are the ultimate source. Bilateral adrenalectomy and dexamethasone administration are associated with greater than 50% reductions of the circulating level of estradiol [9]. The adrenal gland could contribute to the estradiol pool either by direct glandular secretion or by secretion of precursor steroids which are converted peripherally to estradiol. Both estrone and testosterone are converted in the peripheral tissues to estradiol. The finding of a close correlation between estradiol and estrone levels in postmenopausal women suggests that this conversion accounts for most circulating estradiol.

The circulating level of estrone after the menopause is higher than estradiol with most investigators finding a mean concentration of approximately 35 pg/ml [6, 8, 10]. The adrenal gland is the major source of estrone and direct ovarian secretion is minimal. Direct adrenal secretion is minimal. According to the pioneering work of *Siiteri and MacDonald* [11], most estrone is the product of peripheral aromatization of androstenedione. Aromatization of androstenedione has been shown to occur in fat, muscle, liver, kidney, brain, and adrenal glands [12–15]. The conversion has been shown to correlate with body size, heavy women having higher conversion rates and circulating estrogen levels than slender women [8, 16, 17].

Although estrone is the predominant circulating estrogen in menopausal women, estradiol is more biologically potent [18]. The bioavailability of estradiol is dependent upon sex hormone-binding globulin (SHBG) concentrations. SHBG binds a portion of estradiol under physiological conditions and that fraction bound is biologically inactive [19–21]. The remainder of estradiol is bound to albumin (60%) or is unbound (1–3%) [22, 23]. It is theorized that only the absolute free fraction of estradiol is biologically active and that SHBG regulates the percentage of this fraction [24].

SHBG levels have negative correlations with body size. The mechanism for this is unknown but is reversible with weight loss [20, 24–26]. Lower levels of SHBG in heavy subjects have been associated with increased percentages of free estradiol and higher free E_2 levels. Thus, obese women have higher total levels of estrogens due to increased peripheral conversion of adrenal steroids and furthermore have higher levels of free, bioactive estradiol due to lower SHBG levels.

Androgens

During reproductive life the primary ovarian androgen is androstenedione. With the menopause there is a marked reduction of its circulating level from a mean of 1,500 to 900 pg/ml, a level similar to the concentration found in women following oophorectomy [4, 7, 10, 25, 27–29]. The major source of androstenedione in the postmenopausal patients is the adrenal gland. The ovarian contribution to circulating levels of androstenedione is less than 20% in the climacteric patient.

Mean concentration of testosterone in postmenopausal women is 200 pg/ml which is minimally lower than that found in intact ovulatory premenopausal women and distinctly higher than levels observed in premenopausal women following castration [4, 10, 28 32]. The source of circulating testosterone in the postmenopausal patient is ovarian as well as adrenal. The postmenopausal ovary continues to directly secrete testosterone in greater amounts than the premenopausal gonad. This has been supported by ovarian vein sampling studies [33]. Thus, the menopausal ovary has a markedly reduced androstenedione production and a persistent testosterone secretion. This increase in ovarian testosterone secretion coupled with the reduction of estrogen production may explain in part the development of symptoms of defeminization, hirsutism, and even virilism seen in some older women.

Gonadotropins

With the menopause, both luteinizing hormone (LH) and follicle-stimulating hormone (FSH) levels rise substantially. FSH is usually higher than LH due to the slower clearance of FSH from the circulation [33]. Circulating gonadotropins are markedly increased due to the absence of the negative feedback of ovarian steroids on gonadotropin release. The levels of both gonadotropins are not steady but demonstrate periodic oscillation due to the pulsatile release which occurs every 1–2 h. The frequency of the gonadotropin pulses is similar to that seen during the follicular phase of the premenopausal subject. On the other hand, the amplitude is much greater in the postmenopausal patient as a result of increased release of gonadotropin-releasing hormone (GnRH) and enhanced responsiveness of the pituitary to GnRH [34, 35]. Elevated GnRH levels in postmenopausal women are consistent with enhanced hypothalamic activity after ovarian failure [36]. Studies with rhesus monkeys suggest that the source of GnRH is in the arcuate nucleus of the hypothalamus [37, 38].

Physiologic Changes of the Menopause

Hot Flashes

The hot flash is the most common menopausal symptom for which patients seek treatment. In nearly 80% of women, these episodes of perspiration and flushing persist for more than 1 year and in 25–70% they persist for more than 5 years [39–41]. Although the symptoms may persist for an extended period of time, homeostatic adjustments eventually occur in many of the untreated women. It has been commonly stated that hot flashes are more frequent and severe following surgical castration. This thermoregulatory disturbance has been documented in 19 out of 25 women 6 weeks following oophorectomy [42]. The physiologic characteristics of these episodes were similar to those observed after the natural menopause.

Until recently it has been unclear whether hot flashes are due to direct effects of estrogen deficiency or to indirect effects caused by the altered hypothalamic or pituitary function. Recent investigation into the physiology and endocrinology of hot flashes has given new insights into its pathophysiologic mechanisms. *Molnar* [43] has established that the hot flash is a generalized phenomenon with the most notable rises of skin temperature, a reflection of vasodilation, occurring over the fingers and toes. Previously, it had been believed that the physiologic changes were confined to the upper trunk, neck, and face, where women perceived the symptoms most intensely. In a cool ambient environment under basal conditions, continuous recording of finger temperature can be used as an objective marker of the hot flash [44]. Perspiration, the other symptom of the hot flash, is most prominent over the upper body. It can be objectively monitored by continuous measurement of skin resistance over the upper chest [45]. Simultaneous recording of finger temperature, skin resistance, and the onset of subjective symptoms has shown a remarkably consistent and temporal relation among these components. The onset of subjective symptoms is followed in 44 ± 9 s by a rapid fall of skin resistance and in 90 ± 10 s by a rise of skin temperature.

Investigation of the physiologic components of the hot flash and the effects of the resulting heat loss and cooler temperature indicate that the hot flash is a central rather than peripherally mediated disturbance. The combination of cutaneous vasodilation (inhibition of sympathetic noradrenergic tone) and of perspiration (stimulation of sympathetic colonergic tone) cannot be explained on the basis of any currently known peripheral mechanism, but is characteristic of a centrally integrated thermoregulatory response triggered from rostal hypothalamic centers. Furthermore, loss of heat due to peripherally initiated vasodilation and perspiration, leading to fall in core temperature, would result in various homeostatic adjustments to attempt to maintain central temperature. The most prominent of these mechanisms in higher species is behavior. Thus the women would be expected to feel cold and to increase clothing and to move to a warmer location. During the hot flash the behavioral manifestations are exactly opposite, indicating that the mechanism for heat loss is triggered centrally, the core temperature thus being allowed to fall to coincide with a new lower set point [46].

Investigation of the various hormonal components of the hypothalamic pituitary ovarian axis has also yielded information localizing the origin of the hot flash disturbance and elucidating factors that may modulate its occurrence. During continuous monitoring of hot flashes using the objective markers previously noted, blood sampling has shown a striking temporal relation between pulsatile releases of LH and the occurrence of the hot flash [47, 48]. The close relation of the onset of the earliest manifestation of the hot flash with the onset of the LH pulse suggests that either LH or the factors responsible for the pulsatile release of LH are related to the factors triggering the hot flash [49]. Similar relations were not found for circulating estrogens. Further investigation of women with pituitary insufficiency has shown objectively documented hot flashes in the absence of pulsatile release of LH, indicating that LH pulses are merely associated with the phenomenon rather than causing it [50]. Therefore, hypothalamic factors which stimulate the pulsatile release of LH presumably play an integral role in the initiation of the hot flash. The principal hypothalamic center that controls body temperature is located in the anterior hypothalamic and preopic nuclei. One of the main fossi that produce GnRH is also the preoptic nuclei. The three hypothalamic neurotransmitters most strongly linked to GnRH are norepinephrine, dopamine, and opioid peptides. They have all been implicated in the central regulation of body temperature. These neurotransmitters involved in the pulsatile release of GnRH may alter adjacent neurons with thermal regulatory funciton thus activating neuroeffective pathways and initiating heat loss.

The extent of estrogen deficiency differs among postmenopausal women, which may explain why all women do not have hot flashes with the cessation of ovarian function. Extraglandular estrogen production is directly related to body weight and inversely related to circulating concentrations of SHBG [51, 52]. A recent study comparing endogenous estrogen concentrations in women having severe hot flashes with hormone levels in postmenopausal women who have never had the symptom complex has shown lower levels of estrone and estradiol in the symptomatic women. The percent of ideal body weight was significantly lower in the women with hot flashes suggesting that the known effects of body size on estrogen production and plasma-binding protein are significant variables modulating the extent of estrogen deficiency and hypothalamic function [53].

Osteoporosis

Osteoporosis is the most important health hazard associated with the menopause. It is a disorder characterized by a reduction in the quantity of bone without changes in its chemical composition. This process is accelerated by the loss of ovarian function, resulting in a greater prevalence of osteoporosis in women than men [54, 55]. This is a particular problem with early castration and in patients with gonadal dysgenesis. Other factors implicated in the pathogenesis of osteoporosis include immobilization, Caucasian and Oriental race, slender body size, excessive alcohol consumption, low calcium intake, and cigarette smoking. The loss of bone mass produces minimal symptoms but does lead to reduced skeletal strength and fractures. The vertebral body is the most common site of fracture. Fractures of the humerus, distal radius, and upper femur are also enhanced with osteoporosis. The fractured femur is of particular concern. It is associated with appreciable mortality and profound morbidity [56, 57]. Approximately 125,000 hip fractures occurred in older women in the United States in 1979 and this fracture continues to be associated with mortality of approximately 15%. A causal role has been postulated for the calcitropic hormones, parathyroid hormone (PTH), $1,25(OH)_2-D_3$, and calcitonin, in osteoporosis. Studies of PTH and vitamin D have been unable to demonstrate a consistent relationship between levels of these hormones and osteoporosis [58–68]. On the other hand, evidence has accumulated to implicate calcitonin in the pathogenesis of osteoporosis. The main skeletal effect of calcitonin is inhibited bone resorption; the main skeletal defect in osteoporosis is increased bone resorption [69, 70].

Calcitonin and gonadal steroids may be linked in the pathogenesis of osteoporosis. The calcitonin secretion progressively declines with age and is more prominent in women than in men [71, 72]. Animal studies have demonstrated that oophorectomy diminishes calcitonin levels and estradiol administration increases plasma calcitonin. The administration of estrogens has been reported to increase plasma calcitonin in women of all ages [64, 73, 74]. The mechanism of action of estrogen replacement therapy in the treatment of osteoporosis is not clear. The major therapeutic effect of estrogen replacement therapy is to inhibit bone resorption but most investigators have failed to show the presence of estrogen receptors in the bone. Thus estrogens must exert their skeletal effects indirectly perhaps by increasing the plasma calcitonin levels.

Osteoporosis is a disorder of the skeletal system that is at least in part dependent upon the levels of sex hormones and calcemic hormones. Several studies have indicated that low dose estrogen therapy can arrest or retard bone loss if begun shortly after the menopause and studies of estrogen replacement for up to 8 years have reduced the incidence of fractures [75–81]. Studies of longer duration have not been published up to this time.

Cardiovascular Disease

A relationship between the loss of ovarian function and the development of heart disease has been proposed by recent investigations. An autopsy study of American women who had bilateral oophorectomy before the age of 50 indicated that this population has a higher incidence of coronary atherosclerosis, arterial blockage, and myocardial infarction [82]. The Framingham follow-up study of 2,873 women who had biannual examinations for 24 years revealed an increase of heart disease immediately after the menopause [83]. Similar results were reported from Sweden [84]. A study of nonfatal acute myocardial infarction in postmenopausal women found a protective effect of estrogen use [85]. This effect, however, disappeared when other risk factors for myocardial infarction were controlled.

A recent case-controlled study examined estrogen use as reported in medical records from women dying from arteriosclerotic heart disease and matched groups of dead and living controlled subjects. A strong protective effect of estrogens was found [86].

Cessation of ovarian functions is associated with an increase in cardiovascular disease. Furthermore, exogenous estrogen administration in proper doses is instrumental in decreasing the development of cardiovascular disease in the menopausal patient.

Genitourinary Changes

After the menopause, atrophic changes of the vagina occur and are accompanied by symptoms of vaginal dryness, burning, itching, dyspareunia, discharge, and occasional bleeding. Patients may also experience dysuria and urinary frequency in the absence of infection. These urinary symptoms may result from estrogen deficiency, as the urethra and vagina possess a common embryonic origin. Estrogens are effective in overcoming atrophy of the vaginal epithelium and the associated symptoms.

The relief of symptoms of vaginal atrophy occurs with either systemic or vaginally applied estrogen. Contrary to former beliefs, it has been clearly shown that estrogens administered intravaginally enter the blood stream and can reach superphysiologic concentrations [87].

Skin Changes

With aging, noticeable changes occur in the skin. There is generalized thinning accompanied by loss of elasticity which results in wrinkling. The presence of estrogen receptors in certain elements of the skin of mice suggests that estrogens could have direct effect on skin [88]. However, any effects of menopause or estrogen replacement on skin in humans have not been clearly established [89]. Until a beneficial cosmetic effect is shown, the use of estrogens for this indication should not be recommended.

Psychological Changes in Menopause

The psychological characteristics of the menopausal state are incompletely defined. This period of life does not appear to be characterized by a high incidence of new and distinctive mental illness. However, in addition to endocrinologic and physiologic changes, certain depressive-based psychological symptoms can be associated with the menopause. Such symptoms include depressive mood, anxiety, irritability, insomnia, and lack of interest [90].

Despite the severity of such psychic phenomena, very few investigations based on precise experimental data have been carried out to discover the essential pathogenic factors responsible for the onset and the persistence of depressive states during the menopause [91, 92].

The frequency and severity of subjective symptomatology during the menopause are not correlated to the plasma levels of the hormonal secretions most strongly affected by the end of the reproductive cycle [93]. Different levels of gonadotropins, estrogens, progesterone, testosterone, and prolactin do not correspond to the presence or absence of anxious-depressive states or their severity. Thus, it is not the type of severity of endocrinological changes that determines psychic disturbances.

The menopause itself is a biological event marked by hormonal changes together with external factors typical of the menopause, such as change in menstrual flow and physical appearance. This transitional condition may be sufficient to explain the onset of psychological states which affect a certain proportion of the female population. Personality, social, and environmental factors seem to allow sharper differentiation between those women suffering from depressive disturbances and others. The psychopathological picture of the menopausal depressive state has been related to the presence of personality factors of predepressive type (dependence, conventionality, anxiety, and devotion to duty) together with a difficult childhood and a low degree of acceptance of the environment during childhood [94]. Surveys have not shown any consistent association with improvement in performance, mood, or psychological states and estrogen replacement therapy. On the other hand, a prospective double-blind study by *Erlik* et al. [95] has documented an increase in insomnia in postmenopausal women specifically improved by estrogen [95]. Estrogen replacement decreases waking episodes and increases REM sleep. Insomnia was found to be more severe in those postmenopausal women with severe hot flashes which were held responsible for multiple waking episodes as identified by sleep EEGs and hot flash monitoring. This study has suggested that the waking episodes experienced by postmenopausal women were caused by the same central disturbance that is perceived at a cortical level as a hot flash. Part of the improvement of sleep quality by estrogen may be due to the occurrence of fewer waking episodes thereby allowing evolution of sleep to occur in a more normal fashion. Chronic sleep disturbance associated with estrogen deficiency may have secondary effects on other aspects of brain function resulting in anxiety, irritability, and decreased memory [96].

The anxious-depressive syndrome of the menopause is most likely related to a concurrence of a number of factors. Personality and socioenvironmental factors, interaction with endocrinological changes, and alteration in sleep patterns all have a key role in triggering these subjective symptoms.

Treatment of the Menopause

As long as ovarian funciton is sufficient to maintain some uterine bleeding, no treatment is usually required. As the menstrual pattern alters and symptoms commence, patients begin to seek help and their need for treatment must then be addressed.

Every woman with climacteric symptoms deserves an adequate explanation of the physiologic event she is experiencing in order to dispel her fears and minimize symptoms such as anxiety, depression, sleep disturbances, etc. Reassurances should emphasize that the climacteric is not, contrary to anything that she may have heard, a period of sudden aging or personal disaster. Specific reassurance about continued sexual activity is also important.

Estrogen replacement is the hallmark of treatment of the menopause. Although estrogen has been found to be effective in preventing hot flashes, vaginal atrophy, osteoporosis, and coronary artery disease, adverse effects are well recognized. Before administering this form of therapy, a discussion of the advantages as well as the complications and contraindications should be held with each patient. The following is a brief review of the complications.

Complications of Estrogen Therapy

Endometrial Cancer

The importance of estrogens as the cause of endometrial hyperplasia and neoplasia has long been well known. Pathologists have recognized the coexistence of hyperplasia and the apparent evolution of hyperplasia into frank neoplasia [97]. Early studies of women with endometrial cancer showed evidence of estrogen excess including ovarian stromal hyperplasia and high vaginal cornification index. The association of estrogen excess with endometrial cancer is also supported by the observation that obesity (elevated estrone and estradiol levels) in postmenopausal women is a major risk factor for endometrial cancer.

The first case of endometrial cancer occurring in women with long-term use of exogenous estrogens was reported in the early 1960s [98]. Case-controlled studies reported in 1975 showed a uniformly high risk of endometrial cancer associated with estrogen replacement therapy [99–101]. In several reports implicating estrogen usage to endometrial cancer, there is substantial evidence that the association is dose and duration related in respect to estrogen exposure. On the other hand, the addition of a progestogen to the estrogen therapy has been shown to be protective to the endometrium [102]. The prevention of hyperplasia is dependent upon the duration of the progestogen administered each month. Long-term follow-up studies have reported that an 18–32% incidence of hyperplasia with estrogen therapy was significantly reduced to 3–4% with the addition of progestogens for 7 days each month. The lengthening of the duration of the progestogen administration to 10 days reduces the incidence of hyperplasia to 2% and maximum protective effects are obtained with 12–13 days progestogen exposure [103]. The incidence of endometrial cancer with combined estrogen-progestogen regimes is also reduced below that observed in untreated women.

In addition to preventing the development of hyperplasia and carcinoma, progestogens are also capable of reversing spontaneously arising or estrogen-related hyperplasia back to normal endometrium in approximately 95% of cases. These data have been interpreted as providing further evidence that progestin deficiency is one of the major causes of endometrial hyperplasia [104].

Breast Cancer

The breast cancer risk factors of early age at menarche and delayed age at menopause indicate that ovarian estrogen activity is an important determinant of risk to this cancer. This had been strongly supported by findings in the extensive studies of the role of estrogens in the occurrence of mammary tumors in rodents. Early studies of the possible effects of estrogen replacement therapy and the risk of breast cancer were largely follow-up studies without controls. The most credible cohort study to date was performed by *Hoover* et al. [105]. Although they reported only a 25% access risk of breast cancer in their cohort of users of estrogen compared with the general population, they did report a more substantial access among women using high doses for longer duration. *Ross* et al. [106] found an increase in the relative risk of breast cancer for long-term users of oral estrogens. *Gambrell* et al. [107] have recently reported a decreased risk in the development of breast cancer in those postmenopausal women treated with estrogen in combination with progestogens in comparison to an untreated population.

There is significant evidence that estrogen replacement therapy without progestogen is associated with an increased relative risk of breast cancer. The magnitude of the elevated risk is small and has not been consistently found even in the more recent case-control studies. The addition of progestogen to estrogen replacement therapy most likely provides a protective effect on the breat as seen similarly in the uterus.

Liver

Sex steroids have profound effect on hepatic function. Alterations of hepatic protein and lipid metabolism can lead to various other side effects. These include the following:

Hypertension

Hypertension may occur or be exacerbated in women receiving estrogen replacement therapy [108–111]. The elevation of blood pressure is rare and usually reversible when the medication is discontinued. The problem is seen less frequently with estrogen replacement than with the use of oral contraceptives. Although increases of blood pressure have been reported, estrogen replacement therapy has not been associated with an enhanced risk of cerebral vascular accidents [110, 111].

The mechanism responsible for this increase in blood pressure is believed to be related to the renin-angiotensin-aldosterone system [112].

The renin substrate is the rate-limiting step of the renin reaction under physiologic conditions [113]. Estrogen administration stimulates the hepatic synthesis of this protein. Associated with this are increases of angiotensin I and aldosterone.

Thromboembolic Disease

It has been observed that the administration of oral contraceptives increases the risk of overt venous thromboembolic disease and the occurrence of subclinical thrombosis that is extensive enough to be detected by laboratory procedures [114]. In uncontrolled studies, thrombophlebitis has been reported with estrogen replacement therapy, whereas this association has not been found in controlled studies.

Lipids

Estrogen replacement therapy also influences hepatic lipid metabolism. An increased incidence of gallbladder disease has been reported with oral contraceptive usage and estrogen replacement therapy. Small increases of cholesterol which are associated with estrogen replacement therapy can produce precipitation leading to stone formation [115].

Circulating lipids are also influenced by estrogen replacement therapy. Lipids are mostly bound to proteins in the circulation and the concentration of the various types of lipoproteins correlates with the risk of heart disease. Low density to very low density lipoprotein levels correlate positively whereas the high density lipoprotein (HDL) concentrations correlate negatively with the risk of heart disease. Estrogen replacement therapy has been associated with decreases of low density lipoproteins, very low density lipoproteins, and cholesterol and increases of HDL and triglycerides [116, 117]. The effects of estrogen on HDL are blocked with the use of 19 norprogestins (common progestins in the oral contraceptives). The estrogen effect on HDL is not inhibited by the C-21 progestins [118].

Contraindication and Precautions

Contraindications to estrogen replacement therapy include undiagnosed vaginal bleeding, acute liver disease, chronic impaired liver disease, acute vascular thrombosis, neuroopthalmalogic vascular disease, and breast cancer. Estrogen may have adverse effects on some patients with preexisting hypertension, uterine leiomyomata, familial hyperlipodemias, migraine headaches, chronic thrombophlebitis, and gallbladder disease.

Estrogen Replacement Therapy

Every adult woman who develops ovarian failure should be considered for estrogen replacement therapy. Each patient needs to be evaluated individually and her symptoms and risk factors must be considered.

Current replacement therapy should be directed toward the relief of hot flashes, atrophic vaginitis, the prevention of osteoporosis, and the prevention of cardiovascular disease. Its use for other indications should be approached with caution as well-controlled studies supporting additional beneficial effects are lacking.

For hot flashes and vaginal atrophy, the severity of the symptoms is important. If minimal or absent, the need for treatment is reduced. The minimum effective dose required to reduce osteoporosis in postmenopausal women has been determined to be 0.625 mg of conjugated equine estrogens per day. The severity of the hot flash may require higher doses for finite periods of time with progressive reduction in the dose. The prevention of osteoporosis with estrogen requires long-term therapy. High dosage of estrogen in prolonged use has been associated with increased risks of endometrial cancer. Although the addition of progestogen to estrogen replacement therapy has been considered to significantly reduce the risk of endometrial hyperplasia and adenocarcinoma of the uterus, other adverse effects of estrogen therapy are not prevented.

Management of Estrogen Replacement Therapy

Before instituting estrogen replacement therapy for a postmenopausal patient a complete evaluation should be performed. The examination should include a history, specifically referring to the contraindications and precautions of estrogen therapy, and a physical examination including blood pressure, breast examination, and pelvic examination. Following this a careful analysis of the potential benefits and risks of estrogen replacement should be individualized for each patient. If the patient wishes to receive estrogen replacement therapy certain principles should apply.

(1) Estrogen therapy should be given in a cyclical fashion using the lowest dose compatible with the effective treatment of the indicated symptom. Ultimately one should approach the dosage level of 0.625 mg of conjugated estrogens. The medication should be given daily for 3 out of 4 weeks.

(2) The sequential addition of progestogen such as Provera, 10 mg/day, should be administered for 10 days/month regardless of the presence

or absence of the uterus. Recent data have demonstrated a protective effect of progestogens against breast cancer as well as uterine cancer for individuals on estrogen replacement therapy.

(3) Treatment with estrogen and progestogens is instituted without an endometrial biopsy when an individual has not had any postmenopausal bleeding or has significantly irregular perimenopausal bleeding. In light of any postmenopausal bleeding or abnormal perimenopausal bleeding, endometrial biopsy is advocated prior to therapy. This biopsy should be performed in the manner of the vabra or dilatation and curettage. It is recognized that estrogen-progestogen therapy may result in withdrawal vaginal bleeding. If this bleeding occurs at any time other than the expected withdrawal period when no medication is being given, a dilatation and curettage or vabra should be performed. Furthermore, individuals receiving estrogens and progestogen should undergo vabra examinations approximately every 2 years. The presence of endometrial hyperplasia may require discontinuation of the estrogen therapy or more prolonged use of progestogens with careful monitoring.

(4) Patients on estrogen replacement therapy should be seen at 6- to 12-month intervals with frequent monitoring of blood pressure and breast examinations.

Route of Administration

Oral therapy is the preferred route of administration of cyclic estrogens and progestogen therapy despite the association with enhanced hepatic effects. The orally administered hormone is absorbed by the intestine and delivered directly to the liver through the protal circulation. Before entry into the general circulation the administered estrogen exerts effects on hepatic function and also is partially degraded to less active metabolites. Thus the portal concentration of estrogens is 4–5 times higher than the level in general circulation after oral administration.

Injectable therapy, while effective, is not recommended on the basis of cost, dose effectiveness, and the hazards of prolonged action. Vaginal placement is effective for relieving symptoms of atrophy and may also be efficacious in treating other complaints such as osteoporosis with very high doses. It has previously been assumed that estrogen administered vaginally had only topical effects and was not absorbed systemically. However, higher blood concentrations of estrogens are achieved after vaginal administration. Transdermal administration of estrogen has recently been shown to significantly reduce the frequency of hot flashes and vaginal atrophy. There was, however, no substantiation of a reduction in an accelerated bone loss with this route of administration.

There are many women who have severe menopausal symptoms and contraindications to estrogen replacement. Other medications can be utilized and may be helpful. Hydroxyprogesterone acetate and megestrol acetate have been shown to reduce the incidence of hot flashes. Clonidine, an antihypertensive agent, may also be effective but is associated with significant side effects. Sedatives and psychopharmacologic agents have been used to reduce these symptoms but their efficacies have not been studied critically. A variety of nonestrogenic therapeutic modalities including exercise, calcium, calcitonin, vitamin D, and fluorides have been recommended for their prevention of osteoporosis, but to date only calcium supplements and fluorides have been studied prospectively in a double-blind manner and have been shown to be effective. There is no good substitutional therapy for vaginal atrophy. Dyspareunia may be partially relieved by the use of lubricants.

References

1. Ross, G.T.; Vande Wiele, R.L.: The ovaries; in Williams, Textbook of endocrinology, pp. 368–442 (Saunders, Philadelphia 1974).
2. Baker, T.G.: A quantitative and cytological study of germ cells in human ovaries. Proc. R. Soc. Lond. Ser. B. *158:* 417–433 (1963).
3. Costoff, A.; Mahesh, V.B.: Primordial follicles with normal oocytes in the ovaries of postmenopausal women. J. Am. Geriat. Soc. *23:* 193–197 (1975).
4. Abraham, G.E.; Maroulis, G.B.: Effect of exogenous estrogen on serum pregnenolone, cortisol, and androgens in postmenopausal women. Obstet. Gynec., N.Y., *45:* 271–274 (1975).
5. Baird, D.T.; Guevara, A.: Concentration of unconjugated estrone and estradiol in peripheral plasma in nonpregnant women throughout the menstrual cycle, castrate and postmenopausal women and in men. J. clin. Endocr. Metab. *29:* 149–156 (1969).
6. Chakravarti, S.; Collins, W.P.; Forecast, J.D.; Newton, J.R.; Oram, D.H.; Studd, J.W.W.: Hormonal profiles after the menopause. Br. med. J. *ii:* 784–787 (1976).
7. Judd, H.L.: Hormonal dynamics associated with the menopause. Clin. Obstet. Gynec. *19:* 775–788 (1976).
8. Judd, H.L.; Lucas, W.E.; Yen, S.C.: Serum 17β-estradiol and estrone levels in postmenopausal women with and without endometrial cancer. J. clin. Endoc. Metab. *43:* 272–278 (1976).
9. Veldhuis, J.D.; Santen, R.J.; Santner, S.; Davis, B.; Samojlik, E.; Ruby, E.: Unique pharmacologic estrogen deprivation by aminoglutethimide. Proc. 60th Annu. Meet. Endocrine Soc., Miami 1978, p. 201.

10 Greenblatt, R.B.; Colle, M.L.; Mahesh, V.B.: Ovarian and adrenal steroid production in postmenopausal women. Obstet. Gynec., N.Y. *47:* 383–387 (1976).
11 Siiteri, P.K.; Macdonald, P.C.: Role of extraglandular estrogen in human endocrinology; in Greep, Astwood, Endocrinology handbook of physiology, vol. 2, section 1, pp. 615–629 (American Physiological Society, Washington, 1973).
12 Bolt, H.M.; Gobel, P.: Formation of androgens from estrogens by human subcutaneous adipose tissue in vitro. Hormone metabol. Res. *4:* 312–313 (1972).
13 Longcope, C.; Pratt, J.H.; Schneider, S.H.; Fineberg, S.E.: Aromatization of androgens by muscles and adipose tissue in vivo. J. clin. Endocr. Metab. *46:* 146–155 (1978).
14 Nimrod, A.; Ryan, K.J.: Aromatization of androgens by human abdominal and breast fat tissue. J. Clin. Endocr. Metab. *40:* 367–372 (1975).
15 Schindler, A.E.; Ebert, A.; Fredrick, E.: Conversion of androstenedione to estrone by human fat tissue. J. clin. Endocr. Metab. *35:* 627–630 (1972).
16 Grodin, J.M.; Siiteri, P.K.; Macdonald, P.C.: Source of estrogen production in postmenopausal women. J. clin. Endocr. Metab. *36:* 207–214 (1973).
17 Judd, H.L.; Davidson, B.J.; Frumar, A.M.; Shamonki, I.M.; Lagasse, L.D.; Ballon, S.C.: Serum androgens and estrogens in postmenopausal women with and without endometrial cancer. Am. J. Obstet. Gynec. *136:* 859–871 (1980).
18 Gurpide, E.: Enzymatic modulation of hormonal action at the target tissue. J. Toxicol. envir. Health *4:* 249 (1978).
19 Anderson, D.C.: Sex-hormone-binding globulin. Clin. Endocrinol. *3:* 69 (1974).
20 Nisker, J.A.; Hammond, G.L.; Davidson, B.J.; Frumar, A.M.; Takaki, N.K.; Judd, H.L.; Siiteri, P.K.: Serum sex hormone-binding globulin and the percentage of free estradiol in postmenopausal women with and without endometrial carcinoma. Am. J. Obstet. Gynec. *138:* 637 (1980).
21 Heyns, W.: The steroid-binding beta-globulin of human plasma. Adv. Steroid Biochem. Pharmacol. *6:* 59 (1977).
22 Partridge, W.M.; Mietus, L.J.; Frumar, A.M.; Davidson, B.J.; Judd, H.L.: Inverse relationship between the sex hormone-binding globulin level of human serum and the uni-directional clearance of testosterone and estradiol by rat brain. Am. J. Physiol. *263:* E103 (1980).
23 Hammond, G.L.; Nisker, J.A.; Jones, L.A.; Siiteri, P.K.: Estimation of the percent free steroid in undiluted serum by centrifugal ultrafiltration-dialysis. J. biol. Chem. *255:* 5023 (1980).
24 Demoor, P.; Joossens, J.V.: An inverse relation between body weight and the activity of the steroid binding beta globulin in human plasma. Steroidologia *1:* 120 (1970).
25 Vermeulen, A.; Verdonck, L.; Van der Straten, M.; Orie, N.: Capacity of the testosterone-binding globulin in human plasma and influence of specific binding of testosterone on its metabolic clearance rate. J. clin. Endocr. Metab. *29:* 1470 (1979)
26 O'Dea, J.P.K.; Wieland, R.G.; Hallberg, M.C.; Llerena, L.A.; Zorn, E.M.; Genuth, S.M.: Effect of dietary weight loss on sex steroid binding, sex steroids, and gonadotropins in obese postmenopausal women. J. Lab. clin. Med. *93:* 1004 (1979).
27 Calanog, A.; Sall, S.; Gordon, G.G.; Southren, A.L.: Androstenedione metabolism in patients with endometrial cancer. Am. J. Obstet. Gynec. *129:* 553–556 (1977).
28 Judd, H.L.; Lucas, W.E.; Yen, S.S.C.: Effect of oophorectomy on circulating testosterone and androstenedione levels in patients with endometrial cancer. Am. J. Obstet. Gynec. *118:* 793–798 (1974).

29 Vermeulen, A.: The hormonal activity of the postmenopausal ovary. J. clin. Endocr. Metab. *42:* 247–253 (1976).
30 Calanog, A.; Sall, S.; Gordon, G.G.; Olivo, J.; Southren, A.L.: Testosterone metabolism in endometrial cancer. Am. J. Obstet. Gynec. *124:* 60–63 (1976).
31 Lloyd, C.W.; Lobotsky, J.; Barid, D.T.; McCracken, J.A.; Weisz, J.; Pupkin, M.; Zamartu, J.; Puga, J.: Concentration of unconjugated estrogens, androgens, and gestagens in ovarian and peripheral venous plasma of women: the normal menstrual cycle. J. clin. Endocr. Metab. *32:* 155–166 (1971).
32 Vermeulen, A.; Verdonck, L.: Sex hormone concentrations in postmenopausal women. Clin. Endocrinol. *9:* 59–66 (1978).
33 Yen, S.S.C.; Llerena, O.; Pearson, O.H.; Littell, S.: Disappearance rates of endogenous follicle-stimulating hormone in serum following surgical hypophysectomy in man. J. clin. Endocr. Metab. *30:* 235–329 (1970).
34 Santen, R.J.; Bardin, C.W.: Episodic luteinizing hormone secretion in man. J. clin. Invest. *52:* 2617–2628 (1973).
35 Yen, S.S.C.; Tsai, C.C.; Naftolin, F.; Vandenberg, G.; Ajabor, L.: Pulsatal patterns of gonadotropin release in subjects with and without ovarian failure. J. clin. Endocr. Metab. *34:* 671–675 (1972).
36 Bourguiganon, J.; Hoyoux, C.; Reuten, A.; Franchimont, P.: Urinary excretion of immunoreactive luteinizing hormone-releasing hormone-like material and gonadotropins at different stages of life. J. clin. Endocr. Metab. *48:* 78–85 (1979).
37 Krey, L.C.; Butler, W.R.; Knobil, E.: Surgical disconnection of the medial basal hypothalamus and pituitary function in the rhesus monkey. I. Gonadotropin secretion. Endocrinology *96:* 1073–1087 (1975).
38 Plant, T.M.; Krey, L.C.; Moossy, J.; McCormack, J.T.; Hess, D.L.; Knobil, E.: The arcuate nucleus and the control of gonadotropin and prolactin secretion in the female rhesus monkey. Endocrinology *102:* 52–62 (1978).
39 Jaszmann, L.; Van Lith, N.D.; Zaat, J.C.A.: The perimenopausal symptoms. Med. Gynaecol. Sociol. *4:* 268–76 (1969).
40 McKinlay, S.; Jefferys, M.: The menopausal syndrome. Br. J. prev. soc. Med. *28:* 108–115 (1974).
41 Thompson, B.; Hart, S.A.; Durno, D.: Menopausal age and symptomatology in general practice. J. biol. Sci. *5:* 71–82 (1973).
42 DeFazio, J.; Meldrum, D.R.; Lauffer, L.; Vale, W.; Rivier, J.; Lu, J.K.H.; Judd, H.L.: Induction of hot flashes in premenopausal women treated with a long-acting GnRH agonist. J. clin. Endocr. Metab. *56:* 445–448 (1983).
43 Molnar, G.W.: Body temperature during menopausal hot flashes. J. appl. Physiol. *38:* 499–503 (1975).
44 Meldrum, D.R.; Shamonki, I.M.; Frumar, A.M.; Tataryn, I.V.; Chang, R.J.; Judd, H.L.: Elevation in skin temperature of the finger as an objective index of postmenopausal hot flashes: standardization of the technique. Am. J. Obstet. Gynec. *135:* 713–717 (1979).
45 Tataryn, I.V.; Loxax, P.; Bajorek, J.G.; Chesarek, W.; Meldrum, D.R.; Judd, H.L.: Postmenopausal hot flashes: a disorder of thermal regulation. Maturitas *2:*101–107 (1980).
46 Meldrum, D.R.: The pathophysiology of postmenopausal symptoms. Semin. reprod. Endocrinol. *1:* 11–17 (1983).

47 Tataryn, I.V.; Meldrum, D.R.; Lu, K.H.; Frumar, A.M.; Judd, H.L.: LH, FSH and skin temperature during the menopausal hot flash. J. clin. Endocr. Metab. 49: 152–154 (1979).
48 Casper, R.F.; Yen, S.S.C.; Wilkes, M.M.: Menopausal flushes: a neural endocrine link with pulsatile luteinizing hormone secretion. Science 205: 823–825 (1979).
49 Meldrum, D.R.; Tataryn, I.V.; Frumar, A.M.; Erlik, Y.; Lu, J.K.H.; Judd, H.L.: Gonadotropins, estrogens, and adrenal steroids during the menopausal hot flash. J. clin. Endocr. Metab. 50: 685–689 (1980).
50 Meldrum, D.R.; Erlik, Y.; Lu, J.K.H.; Judd, H.L.: Objectively recorded hot flashes in patients with pituitary insufficiency. J. clin. Endocr. Metab. 52: 684–687 (1981).
51 Macdonald, P.C.; Edmond, C.D.; Hemsell, D.L.; Porter, J.C.; Siiteri, P.K.: Effect of obesity on conversion of plasma androstenedione to estrogen in postmenopausal women with or without endometrial cancer. Am. J. Obstet. Gynec. 130: 448–455 (1978).
52 Nisker, J.A.; Hammond, G.L.; Davidson, B.J.: Serum sex hormone-binding globulin capacity and the percentage of free estradiol in postmenopausal women with and without endometrial carcinoma. Am. J. Obstet. Gynec. 138: 637–642 (1980).
53 Erlik, Y.; Meldrum, D.R.; Judd, H.L.: Lower circulation estrogens in postmenopausal women with frequent hot flashes. Obstet. Gynec., N.Y. 59: 403–497 (1982).
54 Albright, F.; Bloomberg, E.; Smith, P.H.; et al.: Postmenopausal osteoporosis. Trans. Ass. Am. Phys. 55: 298 (1940).
55 Jowsey, J.; Phil, D.; Kelly, P.; et al.: Quantitative microradiographic studies of normal and osteoporotic bone. J. Bone Jt Surg. 47A: 785 (1965).
56 Knowleden, J.; Buhr, A.J.; Bunbar, O.: Incidence of fracture in persons over 35 years of age. Br. J. prev. soc. Med. 18: 130 (1964).
57 Meyn, M.A., Jr.; Hopson, C.; Jayasanksar, S.: Fracture of the hip in the institutionalized psychotic patient. Clin. Orthop. 122: 128 (1977).
58 Teitelbaum, S.L.; Rosenberg, E.M.; Richardson, C.A.; Avioli, L.V.: Histological studies of bone from normocalcemic postmenopausal osteoporotic patients with increased circulating parathyroid hormone. J. clin. Endocr. Metab. 42: 537–543 (1976).
59 Parthemore, J.G.; Roos, B.A.; Parker, D.C.; Kripke, D.F.; Deftos, L.J.: Assessment of acute and chronic changes in parathyroid hormone secretion by a radioimmunoassay with predominant specificity for the carboxyterminal region of the molecule. J. clin. Endocr. Metab. 47: 284–289 (1978).
60 Franchimont, P., Heynen, G.: Parathormone and calcitonin in osteoporosis; in Parathormone and calcitonin radioimmunoassay in various medical and osteoarticular disorders, pp.101–107 (Lippincott, Philadelphia 1976).
61 Dequeker, J.; Bouillon, R.: Parathyroid hormone secretion and 25-hydroxyvitamin D levels of primary osteoporosis. Calcif. Tissue Res. 22: 495–296 (1977).
62 Riggs, B.L.; Gallagher, J.C.; Deluca, H.F.; Edis, A.J.; Lambert, P.W.; Arnaud, C.D.: A syndrome of osteoporosis increased serum immunoreactive parathyroid hormone, an inappropriately low serum 1,25-dihydroxyvitamin D. Mayo Clin. Proc. 53: 701–706 (1978).
63 Bouillon, R.; Geusens, P.; Dequeker, J.; Demoore, P.: Parathyroid function in primary osteoporosis. Clin. Sci. mol. Med. 57: 167–171 (1979).
64 Stevenson, J.C.; Abeyasekera, G.; Hillyard, C.J.; et al.: Calcitonin and the calcium-regulating hormones of postmenopausal women: effect of estrogens. Lancet i: 6793–6795 (1981).

65 Gallagher, J.C.; Riggs, B.L.; Jerpbak, C.M.; Arnaud, C.D.: The effect of age on serum immunoreactive parathyroid hormone in normal and osteoporotic women. J. Lab. clin. Med. *95:* 373–385 (1980).

66 Riggs, B.L.; Arnaud, C.D.; Jousey, J.; Goldsmith, R.S.; Kelly, P.J.: Parathyroid function in primary osteoporisis. J. clin. Invest. *52:* 181–184 (1973).

67 Gallagher, J.C.; Riggs, B.L.; Eisman, J.; Jamstra, A.; Arnaud, S.B.; Deluca, H.F.: Intestinal calcium absorption and serum vitamin D metabolites in normal subjects and osteopenic patients. J. clin. Invest. *64:* 729–736 (1979).

68 Okano, K.; Nakai, R.; Harasawa, M.: Endocrine factors in senile osteoporosis. Endocr. Jap. *26:* 23–30 (1979).

69 Nordin, B.E.C.: Treatment of postmenopausal osteoporosis. Drugs *18:* 484–492 (1979).

70 Gordan, G.S.: Drug treatment of the osteoporoses. Annu. Rev. Pharmacol. Toxicol. *18:* 253–268 (1978).

71 Shamonki, I.M.; Frumar, A.M.; Tataryn, I.V.; et al.: Age related changes of calcitonin secretion in females. J. clin. Endocr. Metab. *50:* 437–439 (1980).

72 Deftos, L.J.; Weisman, M.N.; Williams, G.W.; et al.: Influence of age and sex on plasma calcitonin in human beings. New Eng. J. Med. *302:* 1351–1353 (1980).

73 Hillyard, C.J.; Stevenson, J.C.; MacIntyre, I.: Relative deficiency of plasma-calcitonin in normal women. Lancet *i:* 961–962 (1978).

74 Morimoto, S.; Onishi, T.; Okaya, Y.; Tanaka, K.; Tsuji, M.; Kumahara, Y.: Comparison of human calcitonin secretion after a one minute calcium infusion in young, normal and elderly subjects. Endocr. jap. *26:* 207–211 (1979).

75 Lindsay, R.; Hart, D.M.; Aitken, J.M.; et al.: Long-term prevention of postmenopausal osteoporosis by estrogen. Lancet *i:* 1038 (1976).

76 Recker, R.R.; Saville, P.D.; Heaney, R.P.: The effect of estrogens and calcium carbonate on bone loss in postmenopausal women. Ann. intern. Med. *89:* 649 (1977).

77 Horsman, A.; Gallagher, J.; Simpson, M.; et al.: Prospective trial of estrogen and calcium in postmenopausal women. Br. med. J. *ii:* 789 (1977).

78 Nachtigall, L.E.; Nachtigall, R.H.; Nachtigall, R.D.; et al.: Estrogen replacement therapy. I. (A) ten year prospective study in the relationship to osteoporosis. J. Am. Coll. Obstet. Gynec. *53:* 277 (1979).

79 Lindsay, R.; Hart, D.M.; Maclean, A.: Bone response to termination of estrogen treatment. Lancet *i:* 1325 (1978).

80 Hutchinson, T.A.; Polanski, S.M.; Feinstein, A.R.: Postmenopausal estrogens protect against fractures of hip and distal radius. A case controlled study. Lancet *ii:* 705 (1979).

81 Weiss, N.C.; Ure, C.L.; Ballard, J.H.: Decreased risk of fractures of the hip and lower forearm with postmenopausal use of estrogen. New Engl. J. Med. *303:* 1195 (1980).

82 Parrish, H.M.; Carr, C.A.; Hall, D.G.; King, T.M.: Time interval from castration and premenopausal women to development of excessive coronary atherosclerosis. Am. J. Obstet. Gynec. *99:* 155–162 (1967).

83 Gordon, T.; Kannel, W.B.; Hjortland, M.C.; McMamara, P.M.: Menopause and coronary heart disease: the Framingham study. Ann. intern. Med. *89:* 157–161 (1978).

84 Bengtsson, C.: Ischemic heart disease in women. Acta med. scand., suppl. 549, pp. 75–81 (1973).

85 Rosenberg, L.; Armstrong, D.; Jick, H.: Myocardial infarction and estrogen therapy in postmenopausal women. New Engl. J. Med. *294:* 1256–1259 (1976).

86 Ross, P.K.; Paganini-Hill, A.; Mack, T.M.; Arthur, M.; Henderson, B.E.: Menopausal estrogen therapy in protection from death, from ischemic heart disease. Lancet *i:* 858–860 (1981).
87 Riggs, L.A.; Hermann, H.; Yen, S.S.C.: Absorption of estrogens from vaginal creams. New Engl. J. Med. *298:* 195–197 (1978).
88 Stumpf, W.E.; Sar, M.; Joshi, S.G.: Estrogen target cells in the skin. Experientia *30:* 196–198 (1974).
89 Shahrad, P.; Marks, R.: A pharmacological effect of estrone on human epidermis. Br. J. Derm. *97:* 383–386 (1977).
90 Brown, M.C.: The management of the menopause and postmenopause years; in Campbell (MTP, Lancaster 1976).
91 Hertz, D.G.; Steiner, J.E.; Zuckermann, H.; Pazanti, S.: Psychosomatics: 1974, 1971.
92 Schneider, M.A.; Brotherton, P.L.; Hailes, J.: Med. J. Aust. *30:* 162 (1977).
93 Castrogiovanni, P.; Brunori Deluca, I.; Teti, G.; Corradi, I.; Moggs, G.; Zecca, R.; Murru, S.; Silvestri, D.; Fioretti, P.: Depressive states during the menopause: a preliminary study of endocrinological, socio-environmental, and personality factors; in Fioretti, Martini, Melis, Yen. The menopause: clinical endocrinological and pathophysiological aspects, p. 475 (Academic Press, New York 1982).
94 Cassano, G.B.; Castrogiovanni, P.: S.A.D.-Scala di autovalutazione per la depressione (International Committee for Prevention and Treatment of Depression, 1977).
95 Erlik, Y.; Tataryn, I.V.; Meldrum, D.R.; Lomax, P.; Bajorek, J.G.; Judd, H.L.: Association of waking episodes with menopausal hot flashes. J. Am. med. Ass. *245:* 1741–1744 (1981).
96 Campbell, S.; Whitehead, M.: Estrogen therapy in the postmenopausal syndrome. Clin. Obstet. Gynec. *4:* 31–37 (1977).
97 Sommers, S.C.; Meissner, W.A.: Endocrinologic abnormalities accompanying human endometrial cancer. Cancer *10:* 516–521 (1957).
98 Gusberg, S.B.; Hall, R.E.: Precursors of corpus cancer. III. The appearance of cancer of the endometrium in estrogenically conditioned patients. Obstet. Gynec., N.Y. *17:* 397–412 (1961).
99 Smith, D.C.; Prentice, R.; Thompson, D.J.; Herrmann, W.L.: Association of exogenous estrogen and endometrial carcinoma. New Engl. J. Med. *293:* 1164–1167 (1975).
100 Ziel, H.K.; Finkle, W.D.: Increased risk of endometrial carcinoma among sers of conjugated estrogens. New Engl. J. Med. *293:* 1167–1170 (1975).
101 Mack, T.M.; Pike, M.C.; Henderson, B.E.; et al.: Estrogens and endometrial cancer in a retirement community. New Engl. J. Med. *294:* 1262–1267 (1976).
102 Whitehead, M.I.; King, R.J.B.; McQueen, J.; Campbell, S.: Endometrial histology in biochemistry in climateric women during estrogen and estrogen-progesteron therapy. J. R. Soc. Med. *72:* 322 (1979).
103 Studd, J.W.W.; Thom, M.H.; Paterson, M.E.L.; Wade-Evans, T.: The prevention and treatment of endometrial pathology in postmenopausal women receiving endogenous estrogens; in Pasetto, Paoletti, Ambrus, The menopause and postmenopause, pp. 127–139 (MTP Press, Lancaster 1980).
104 Gambell, R.D.: Clinical use of progestins in the menopausal patient. J. reprod. Med. *27:* 131 (1982).
105 Hoover, R.; Gray, L.A.; Cole, M.; MacMahon, B.: Menopausal estrogen in breast cancer. New Engl. J. Med. *295:* 401–405 (1976).

106 Ross, R.K.; Paganini-Hill, A.; Gerkins, V.R.; et al.: A case-control study of menopausal estrogen therapy in breast cancer. J. Am. med. Ass. *243:* 1635–1639 (1980).
107 Gambrell, D.R.; Maier, R.; Sanders, B.I.: Decreased incidence of breast cancer in postmenopausal estrogens-progestogen users. Obstet. Gynec., N.Y. *62:* 435–443 (1983).
108 Crane, M.G.; Harris, J.J.; Winsor, W.: Hypertension oral contraceptive agents, and conjugated estrogens. Ann. intern. Med. *74:* 13–21 (1971).
109 Stern, M.P.; Brown, B.W.; Haskell, W.L.; Farquhar, J.W.; Wehrle, C.L.; Wood, P.D.S.: Cardiovascular risk and use of estrogens or estrogen-progestogenic combinations. J. Am. med. Ass. *235:* 811–815 (1976).
110 Pfeffer, R.I.; Van den Noort, S.: Estrogen use and stroke risk in postmenopausal women. Am. J. Epidem. *103:* 445–446 (1976).
111 Pfeffer, R.I.: Estrogen use, hypertension and stroke in postmenopausal women. J. chron. Dis. *31:* 389–398 (1978).
112 Laragh, J.H.; Sealey, J.E.; Ledingham, J.G.; Newton, M.A.: Oral contraceptives: renin, aldosterone and high blood pressure. J. Am. med. Ass. *201:* 918–922 (1967).
113 Weirr, J.; Briggs, E.M.; Mack, A.; et al.: Blood pressure in women after one year of oral contraception. Lancet *i:* 467–470 (1971).
114 Vassey, M.P.: Female hormones and vascular disease: epidemiologic overview. Br. J. Family Planning *6:* 1–12 (1980).
115 Small, D.M.: The etiology and pathogenesis of gallstones. Adv. Surg. *10:* 63–85 (1966).
116 Bradley, T.T.; Wingerd, J.; Petitti, D.B.; Krauss, R.M.; Ramcharan, S.: Serum high density lipoprotein cholesterol and women using oral contraceptives, estrogens and progestins. New Engl. J. Med. *299:* 17–20 (1978).
117 Wallace, R.B.; Hoover, J.; Barrett-Connor, E.; et al.: Altered plasma lipid and lipoprotein levels associated with oral contraceptive in estrogen use. Lancet *ii:* 11–14 (1979).
118 Hirvonen, C.; Milkonen, M.; Manninen, V.: The effective different progestins on lipoproteins during postmenopausal replacement therapy. New Engl. J. Med. *304:* 560 (1981).

John DeFazio, MD, Department of Obstetrics and Gynecology, Case Western Reserve University School of Medicine, Division of Reproductive Endocrinology and Infertility, University Hospitals of Cleveland, Cleveland, OH 44106 (USA)

Female Sexuality and Feminine Development: Freud and His Legacy

L. M. Lothstein

Department of Psychiatry, Case Western Reserve University, University Hospitals of Cleveland, Ohio, USA

Introduction

The decade of the 1970s was an explosive one in terms of research and reformulations of theories of femininity and female sexuality [24, 26, 28, 34]. *Freud's* [10–12] pioneering views on these subjects, which had dominated clinical thinking, were, for the first time, subjected to serious theoretical and empirical challenges. Even conservative psychoanalysts as *Stoller* [37] viewed *Freud's* original views on women as a 'strange definition of feminity'. Indeed, *Freud's* theories of female sexuality and femininity were transformed, revised, and in many instances discarded. A new wave of theories and research on femininity and female sexuality were swept into the public domain (largely as a result of the media's preoccupation with reporting the politics and polemics of radical feminists and political activists whose intent was to restructure society's negative view of women). Indeed, it appeared that only a revolutionary viewpoint could nudge a conservative society away from its complacent view of women as dependent, passive, masochistic, and inferior.

In this paper I will examine *Freud's* hypotheses about femininity and female sexuality in light of recent empirical and observational research on the early childhood development of women and the newer conceptualizations of female sexuality which have evolved from that research. Finally, I will address those issues as they may have bearing on the daily practice of the obstetrician-gynecologist and other medical specialists whose target population are women.

Freud's View on Female Sexuality and Femininity

Freud viewed each woman as establishing her femininity and female sexuality on a masculine base. That is, *Freud* viewed the original state of all girls as 'male'. Equating the clitoris with the phallus, *Freud* viewed the little girl's sexual organ as a 'little penis' and that, according to a woman's anatomy and genital aims, 'the little girl is in all respects a little man'. Up until the phallic period, age 3, the development of boys and girls was viewed as parallel. *Freud* did not believe that the little girl was able to mentally represent her vagina until adolescence. Therefore, throughout her childhood the little girl was seen as viewing her genital organ as equivalent to a penis but smaller (and therefore inadequate and inferior to the male's). During a girl's 3rd year, when she became aware of the anatomical distinction between the sexes, *Freud* believed that the little girl finally acknowledged that she is not a little boy, and that she had an inferior sex organ. It was therefore the girl's awareness of her genital inferiority which aroused her anxiety. The end result was that girls were seen as viewing their femaleness as based on genital inferiority, penis envy, profound feelings of inadequacy, heightened castration anxiety, object loss, and a passive, masochistic adaption. Indeed, *Freud* would have us believe that it was the girl's awareness of her penisless state that inaugurated her femininity. That is, a girl's femininity, female core gender identity, and female sexuality were seen as formed as a defense against her castration anxiety; not as the result of a naturally unfolding process involving biological processes and parental, social, and cultural communications about femininity and female sexuality (especially as related to her parents' pleasure in her libidinal attachment to a female body).

In order to achieve her femininity, *Freud* stated that every girl had to pass from a masculine to a feminine phase of development. That is, she had to switch her primary erogenous zone from the clitoris (the quasi-penis) to the vagina; to transfer her love object from the mother to the father; and to shift from a negative oedipal relationship with the father (that is, a homosexual relationship) to a positive one. *Freud* believed that since boys did not have to make all these switches, it was more difficult for the girl to achieve her femininity than for a boy to achieve his masculinity. What we know today suggests just the opposite [30, 31].

Some of the consequences of a girl's early relationship to her mother were viewed as predisposing her to homosexuality; with the discovery of her being castrated leading to the initiation of her oedipal complex.

Eventually a girl might despise her mother for depriving her of what she assumed to be her natural birthright, that is, a penis. The attachment to the mother was seen as ending in hate (basically an unconscious reaction).

In summary, *Freud* viewed a girl's femininity as the outcome of a predetermined defensive process in which a girl's femininity and female sexuality were not guaranteed. Indeed, *Freud* held the view that many girls failed to achieve their femininity and female sexuality and developed either a sexual inhibition, a neurosis, or a masculinity complex. The fact that many girls survived this battle for their femininity and female sexuality, and developed a typical female gender identity, is a mystery [22].

Many of *Freud's* contemporaries criticized his views of femininity and female sexuality. Indeed, his theories were immediately attacked by a number of colleagues. Feminist analysts, including *Karen Horney* [16] and *Helene Deutsch* [4], critically challenged *Freud's* views of women as an 'homme manque' what *Jones* [18] summarized 'as a permanently disappointed creature struggling to console herself with secondary substitutes alien to her nature.' Subsequently, feminists [2] have made a frontal assault on *Freud's* patriarchal and phallocentric views of women [1, 32]; views which were based on his acceptance of a specific cultural view of women which molded his thinking about femininity and female sexuality [1]. Recently, outcome studies, from birth onwards, have not only challenged *Freud's* views of women but have suggested an entirely different model of femininity and female sexuality [8, 9, 20, 21, 24, 28].

In summary, while researchers are indebted to *Freud* for his pioneering insights and his struggle to make conceptual sense out of diverse and often confusing material, no one today can seriously defend his view of women (though his psychoanalytic methodology still survives as a powerful conceptual method for exploring the human psyche). Subsequent empirical research into early childhood behavior has challenged *Freud's* views and led to reconceptualizations, reformulations, and revisions of his theory of female sexual development.

New Conceptualizations of Femininity and Female Sexuality

The major challenges to *Freud's* conceptualizations of femininity and female sexuality were based on empirical evidence and observational studies of girls from birth through the 3rd year (when core female gender identity is established). The results of these studies [20, 27, 31] suggest that even by the 3rd year of life 'a little girl is very much a girl and knows it' [21]. That is, a state of primary femininity exists in which naturally occurring feminine behaviors (which are not defensive and non-conflictual) are evident, in some cases even in the 1st year of life. The conclusions, which were arrived at from observational studies on the effects of family communication patterns on a girl's femininity and female sexuality, suggest that a girl's female sexuality and femininity are not established on a masculine base. In effect, the original state of all girls is not male or female but bisexual.

The roots of feminization and female sexuality are structuralized prior to birth and manifested in the parental and family wishes, fantasies, and expectations of the gender of their child-to-be. The unconscious wishes of the parents and grandparents create a favorable or unfavorable environment for the girl who becomes a container of these gender fantasies. The disappointment of a parent who longs for a male child is communicated to the child and may have a devastating effect on the girl's nascent female sexuality and femininity, perhaps sealing her fate by masculinizing her and leading to sexual inhibitions, a neurosis, or masculinity complex. Some of these girls may even become transsexual, other homosexual.

Another significant challenge to *Freud's* hypotheses about femininity and female sexuality suggests that *Freud* erred in viewing the clitoris as an anatomically male organ [8, 36]. Although there are certain functional similarities between the penis and clitoris, they are qualitatively distinct organs and should not be equated either in function or structure. Viewing the clitoris as a qualitatively distinct organ (not as an inferior penis) enables the clinician to formulate a psychology of femininity and female sexuality that is not based on defensive adaptations, genital inferiority, castration anxiety, and penis envy. Such an approach provides a new positive approach for researchers to investigate female sexuality and femininity.

Freud's view that young girls lacked a mental representation of a vagina to provide her childhood experience with 'the center for a feminine gender identity' has also undergone considerable revision. *Roiphe and Galenson* [31] have shown that girls do indeed have a mental representation of their vaginas and an awareness of their genital organs at an extremely early age. This awareness comes from masturbation practices which are carried out at a much earlier age than *Freud* noted. Indeed, a girl's masturbation provides her with a focus for intense pleasure and self-absorption (with the vagina and clitoris as the bodily focus of excitement) which is hypothesized to have a mental representation. In this vein, *Roiphe and Galenson* [31] have postulated that during the 2nd year of life an early genital phase occurs. During this time frame girls already show evidence of having a mental representation of their vagina (as evidenced by their memory to explore their vaginal areas and stimulate their clitoris). Even before *Roiphe and Galenson's* [31] discovery, analysts, personally and clinically, took issue with *Freud's* ideas which seemed to have been put forward with very little clinical evidence.

Another line of research has even questioned whether a girl needs a vagina in order to consolidate a core female gender identity. *Money and Ehrhardt* [28] have presented evidence that girls born without vaginas are able to establish a typical female core gender identity. In this sense, the feminine self-representation is evident even in girls without a vagina. Moreover, *Freud's* view that the vagina was the more 'mature' female sex organs has also been experimentally challenged by *Masters and Johnson* [25]. Their research has challenged *Freud's* view that the vaginal orgasm represented a higher emotional level than the clitoral orgasm. In effect, *Masters and Johnson* [25] suggested that the most intense orgastic feelings were associated with clitoral masturbation and that the clitoris, rather than the vagina, ought to be viewed as the women's main sexual organ.

Freud's view that a girl's close relationship to her mother would predispose her to homosexuality (and therefore impair her femininity and female sexuality) has also been discredited. It is now believed that the girl's prolonged preoedipal attachment to the mother predisposes her to crises around her self-identity and separateness from mother, not a fear that she will become homosexual [9]. Rather a woman may fear that by merging with mother she will not be able to establish a separate identity and a cohesive self-system. This is an important area for future research and a special area of vulnerability for women.

Freud's confusion between gender identity and sexual preference has also been superceded by newer conceptualizations in which these two lines of thinking are separated. Indeed, one's sexual preference is now viewed as developing along divergent lines to one's gender identity and role.

The most significant developments in our changing concepts of femininity and female sexuality have come about as a result of empirical studies in which family patterns of communication have been observed and investigated. These studies have revealed how patterns of communications and meaning about gender identity and role are transmitted from parent to child.

It is now believed that a primary stage of femininity exists in which the little girl evolves a sense of her femininity and female sexuality even prior to the phallic stage. According to *Kleeman* [21], even by age 3 a 'girl is very much a girl and knows it'. This early stage of primary femininity has been conceptualized by *Stoller* [37] as the result of a complex communicative interchange between the parent and child around the child's evolving gender identity. To the extent that the parents raise their daughter according to her female sex of assignment, and react with pleasurable delight to her emerging femininity and female sexuality, their daughter will be able to evolve a typical femininity, female gender identity and role, and female sexuality. This early period of gender identity (which crystallizes during the second half of the 2nd year of life) involves a complex process of innate behaviors, learned responses, and constitutional issues. All a causal observer may see (even by 18 months of age) is a feminine appearing girl. In some unusual instances in which a young boy's gender identity and role are transposed (that is the young boy has an intense preoccupation with mimicking girls and is obsessed with the idea of becoming a girl), the boy may also exhibit what is called primary femininity [37].

In order to consolidate the rudiments of a core female gender identity in their daughter, parents must empathically relate to their daughter's emerging femininity and female sexuality in a positive and pleasurable way; supporting her budding female core gender identity and role and enabling her to take pride in her evolving female body. Unless the girl takes pride in her female body (and anticipates with joyfulness the eventual growth of breasts) she will be unable to evolve a normal and healthy body image and schema necessary for the establishment of a typical female core gender identity. For girls born without vaginas it is critical that the parents receive support and guidance about how important it is to respond positively to their daughter's female body so that she may evolve a healthy and normal female sexuality and femininity.

By establishing an appropriate 'holding environment' the parents allow their daughter's nascent female self-system to develop and mature so that stable ego mechanisms may also evolve and her gender-self-representational system (especially as it focuses on her core gender identity) may develop normally. We now believe that the precursors of core gender identity involve a typical developmental sequence. This sequence includes the establishment of self-object differentiation, the development of ego mechanisms regulating object and self constancy (especially related to gender issues), and the formation of a female gender-self-representation which coalesces over time into a unity which we label as a girl's core gender identity (an identity that evolves over her lifetime). This identity, which is first noted prior to the child's 3rd birthday, evolves in a developing self-system in which a number of other processes are also developing. These include:

(1) the child's developing the capacity to differentiate her self-object representations;

(2) her ability to separate her self-representation from mother;

(3) the establishment of her ego mechanisms regulating self and object constancy;

(4) the child's libidinal attachment to her body and body image and a sense of pleasure in her femininity and female sexuality;

(5) the development of the capacity for semisymbolic processes of reasoning;

(6) a struggle with their mothers who must allow their daughters to separate, individuate, and establish a separate sense of self;

(7) the psychological issues related to toilet training such as autonomy, control, will, and separateness;

(8) undergoing an early genital phase, which involves intense castration anxiety and a sense of object loss and negativism;

(9) becoming aware of the anatomical distinction between the sexes;

(10) revealing a stage of primary femininity;

(11) beginning to progressively differentiate her body image and schema;

(12) developing a nuclear self-system while establishing her core female gender identity.

In addition to these developmental processes the girl and her environment contribute a special force which shapes and directs her evolving femininity and female sexuality. These include her physical attractiveness and health; her cognitive abilities and overall ego functioning; the birth of a new sibling and her sibling status; losses, separations, abandonments, and deaths; the total effects of her caretakers and peers on helping to facilitate her femininity and female sexuality, and finally, all the nonpredictable environmental impingements which may alter the course of her femininity and female sexuality.

There is clear evidence that during the second half of the 2nd year of life the young girl is busily at work forming a stable female gender-self-representation. This gender-self-representation becomes the focus for her developing femininity and female sexuality. That is, her gender-self-representation forms the primitive nucleus for the girl's nuclear self-system. *Fast* [8] has argued that when viewed within this new empirical framework, *Freud's* ideas of a girl's penis envy and feelings of genital inferiority take on a new interpretation. It is not that a girl becomes devastated when she becomes aware of the anatomical distinction between the sexes and discovers she is not a male (that is, lacks a penis). This interpretation is too concrete and fails to take into account the employment of 'penis envy' as a developmental metaphor [14] and not a literal experience. *Fast* [9] sees the little girl's discovery that boys are sexually different as leading to the conclusion that 'not all sex and gender possibilities (were) open to her'. This interpretation analyzes the girl's reaction as related primarily to separation-individuation phenomena and not just to intense penis envy, castration anxiety, jealousy, and disappointment about her awareness of not having a male genital.

As a phenomenon, penis envy does seem to exist but plays a different role from that which *Freud* noted. Penis envy seems to come into play sometime after the phallic period during a phase labeled as secondary femininity (in which the defensive factors that *Freud* noted now reach ascendancy). But their influence occurs after primary femininity and core gender identity have evolved. When the little girl becomes aware of the anatomical distinction between the sexes around age 3 (during the early genital phase), she may also experience castration anxiety but her interpretation of the event must be reconsidered in light of her cognitive developmental level and her separation-individuation phenomena. The critical factor for the girl is her recognition that 'not all sex and gender possibilities (are) open to her'. This recognition forms the critical mass for developing her femininity and female sexuality and the narcissistic vulnerabilities associated with her female gender identity. Ultimately a girl's femininity and female sexuality are the result of an active developmental progression of her self-system and core gender identity (and not the result of a defensive process). In the end the little girl's gender identity and role almost appear as if they developed by sleight of hand, as if they were imprinted on her, rather than evolving out of biological, social, familial, psychological processes which are in a constant state of change.

The Psychobiological Sphere

Another line of research into female sexuality and femininity focuses on studies in behavioral endocrinology [28] and the way in which prenatal hormones influence postnatal behavior. Some researchers [15] have even postulated that there is a critical period during fetal development in which neuronal pathways organizing male and female brain development are established (suggesting that males and females have differently organized brains). In support of this idea, *Money and Ehrhardt* [28] have discovered that childhood and adult sex stereotypical behaviors are organized and activated by the effects of intrauterine sex-specific hormones. For example, girls whose intrauterine environment was contaminated by androgens revealed behavioral patterns during latency (ages 6–11) which were characteristically tomboyish. These girls showed a preference for boys' play, engaged in rough and tumble play, preferred utilitarian clothing (to the frilly clothing of girls), were athletic, and experienced a higher sex drive than same sex agemates who were not prenatally primed as 'males'. However, as adults very few of these girls became homosexual. Even during childhood these girls reported heterosexual imagery and wishes to get married and have children. They knew that they were females and had no desire to change sex. While the results of these studies suggest the possibility of a biological basis for some forms of 'tomboyish' behavior in girls, it is clear that the girl's erotic imagery was heterosexual and none of the girls studied doubted that they were females. Summarizing the findings of the effects of prenatal hormones on gender identity, *Ehrhardt and Meyer-Bahlburg* [5] concluded that 'the evidence accumulated so far suggests that human psychosexual differentiation is influenced by prenatal hormones, albeit to a degree... The development of gender identity seems to depend largely on the sex of rearing'.

In addition to the effects of prenatal hormones on behavior, *Money and Ehrhardt* [28] have also investigated how diverse hormonal processes may profoundly affect a girl's gender identity (e.g. progentin-induced hermaphroditism, female adrenogenital syndrome, and postnatal androgenization). For example, in girls born with adrenogenital syndrome the effects of masculinization may be counteracted by appropriate drug replacement therapy. However, a number of girls with adrenogenital syndrome born before 1950 (prior to the discovery of medication to treat their condition) were eventually raised as boys. It appears that the effect of excessive androgens on females is to influence a girl's gender development by providing both the girl and her parents with confusing information about how they should be sexually assigned and reared.

Another area of interest has focused on the relationship between the effects of chromosomal abnormalities on femininity and female sexuality.

A majority of the studies in this area have investigated girls with Turner's syndrome (a gender defect), who had short stature, appeared male, were infertile, and exhibited psychosexual immaturity [28]. In spite of their chromosomal abnormalities these girls were eventually able to differentiate a female gender identity. These findings suggest that the effects of the sex of assignment at birth, and the sex in which a child was reared are the critical factors in a girl's gender identity differentiation and not her chromosomal or hormonal sex.

One study [17] which challenges *Money and Ehrhardt's* [28] environmental hypothesis of female gender identity reported on 38 cases of Dominican male children who were raised as girls but who were later diagnosed as having a rare genetically determined enzyme deficiency (delta 4-steroid 5-alpha-reductase). Eventually, when these 'girls' were between the ages of 7 and 12, they changed their gender to male without any apparent difficulty. The enzyme deficiency affected their genital appearance so that they were raised as girls though they 'knew' they were boys and were not surprised when they began to develop as boys at puberty. The fact that the children had little difficulty adjusting to the new role was attributed to the fact their Dominican culture had a mechanism to explain their condition and accept their gender transformation. While this study is quite intriguing, the results have not been duplicated either by other investigators or in other cultures [29].

Another area of investigation focuses on the relationship between organic brain deficits, including temporal lobe disorders, and the effects on female sexuality and feminine development [3, 7]. While several female transsexuals have been demonstrated to have temporal lobe disorders and abnormal EEG pathology [3, 7], there is also preliminary evidence that certain drugs may play an activating, if not organizing role in gender role and identity disorders [23].

Several studies [19, 33] have also focused on the relationship between increased androgen levels in women and the effects on one's female sexuality and femininity (some of these findings have been related to the effects of physical disease such as Stein-Leventhal syndrome, Cushing's syndrome, etc.). While these findings are preliminary, they suggest that the extent to which an adult female's gender identity will be threatened by an acquired adult disease is directly related to her earlier foundation of her gender identity and role. That is, the effects of physical disease are to activate a preexisting organized pattern of female sexuality and femininity.

More recently investigators have focused on how H-Y antigen factor [35] may contribute to a woman's sexuality and gender identity. While much of the H-Y antigen research has focused on issues related to female transsexualism [6], some investigators are trying to show how H-Y antigen may be the 'mysterious' biological substrate of female (or male) sexuality and femininity.

In yet another attempt to challenge the environmental hypothesis *Stoller* [38] reported on a woman with a life-long gender identity disorder whom he saw over a 27-year period. The woman was described as having 'an incessant drive towards masculinity'. Eventually she turned out to have a rare hormone enzyme defect (17β-hydroxysteroid dehydrogenase deficiency) which caused her anatomic hermaphroditism. While cases such as this one point to the importance of keeping an open mind about the possible biological underpinnings of one's gender identity and role, no conclusive evidence is provided that her condition was solely biological. In summary, the psychobiological research into female sexuality and femininity contraindicates *Freud's* hypothesis that 'anatomy is destiny'. The origins of female sexuality and femininity are now viewed in a much broader perspective in which a number of social, psychological, and cultural factors are seen as playing dominant roles in their development. In addition, genes, chromosomes, enzymes, neurotransmitters, neurohormones, prenatal hormones, and H-Y antigens are also viewed as contributing to the final form of female sexuality and femininity. However, these biological factors play a secondary role to social learning factors in the formation of gender identity. Indeed, little has changed in the last 30 years and researchers still believe that it is the sex that the child is assigned at birth and the sex of rearing that seem to be the critical and determining factors in the establishment of a girl's core female gender identity. In this sense, the views of *Money* et al. [27] that gender identity and role are determined predominately by the sex of assignment and rearing of the child, have been corroborated.

Implications for the Medical Practitioner

Clearly the newer developments in female sexuality and femininity make it imperative that physicians familiarize themselves with these concepts and findings in order to educate their female patients about typical female sexual and gender development. Once the physician is able to identify the normal developmental sequence from primary femininity, core gender identity, early genital phase, to secondary femininity, the physician will be better able to counsel his female patients about how their emotional development secondary to gender development may affect their physical and emotional well-being. These new concepts of female sexuality and femininity ought to lead to new conceptualizations of psychosomatic and somatopsychic illness.

Those girls who failed to show signs of evolving a core female gender identity (by age 2) must be viewed as at high risk for serious emotional disorders. That is, the little girl who disavows her body, attempts to mutilate herself, and rejects her female body is especially at high risk for becoming gender dysphoric (perhaps transsexual). Physicians must realize that girls with severe gender identity pathology do not outgrow their disorder. As opposed to tomboyism, which often disappears in adolescence, girls do not outgrow severe gender identity disorders. Female patients with severe gender identity disorders should not be advised that they will outgrow their disorder. Psychotherapy is the treatment of choice.

While there is a wealth of evidence suggesting a possible biological underpinning to one's gender identity, the evidence strongly supports an environmental hypothesis. That is, a child's gender identity is primarily the result of the sex of rearing and the sex of assignment. For those women with female offspring who have an intersexual disorder or hermaphroditism, the physician (especially the obstetrician-gynecologist) is in a prime position to educate the family members about what they may expect in terms of behaviors and how they may best relate to their daughters by positively reinforcing her femininity and female sexuality. For those women who have children with primarily functional gender pathology the physician can suggest ways in which the parents may communicate their pleasure in their daughter's female sexuality and femininity. Acting in this capacity the physician can help to dispel myths about female sexuality and femininity and create a viable atmosphere for parents to raise girls who are devoid of certain sexual inhibitions, neuroses, and masculinity complexes.

References

1   Breger, L.: Freud's unfinished jouney (Routledge & Kegan, London 1981).
2   Chesler, P.: Women and madness (Doubleday, Garden City 1972).
3   Davies, B.; Morgenstern, F.: A case of cysticercois, temperoal lobe epilepsy and transvestism. J. Neurol. *23:* 247–249 (1960).

4   Deutsch, H.: The psychology of women (Grune & Stratton, New York 1944).
5   Ehrhardt, A.; Meyer-Bahlburg, H.: Effects of prenatal sex hormones on gender related behavior. Science *211:* 1312–1317 (1981).
6   Eicher, W.: Transsexualism and H-Y antigen; in Pauly, Abstr. Proc. 7th Int. Gender Dysphoria Ass. (University of Nevada, Reno 1981).
7   Epstein, A.: Relationship of fetishism and transvestism to brain and particularly to temporal lobe dysfunction. J. nerv. ment. Dis. *133:* 247–253 (1961).
8   Fast, I.: Developments in gender identity: the original matrix. Int. Rev. Psycho-Anal. *5:* 265–273 (1978).
9   Fast, I.: Developments in gender identity: Gender differentiation in girls. Int. J. Psycho-Analysis. *60:* 443–453 (1979).
10 Freud, S.: Some psychical consequences of the anatomical distinction between the sexes; standard ed., vol. *19,* pp. 248–258 (Hogarth Press, London 1961).
11 Freud, S.: Female sexuality; standard ed., vol. *21,* pp. 233–243 (Hogarth Press, London 1961).
12 Freud, S.: Femininity; standard, ed., vol. *22,* pp. 112–135 (Hogarth Press, London 1961).
13 Breenson, R.: Dis-identifying from mother. Int. J. Psycho-Analysis *49:* 370–374 (1968).
14 Grossman, W.; Stewart, W.: Penis envy: from childhood wish to developmental metaphor. J. Am. psychoanal. Ass. *24:* 193–212 (1976).
15 Hines, M.: Prenatal gonadal hormones and sex differences in human behavior. Psychol. Bull. *92:* 56–80 (1982).
16 Horney, K.: Feminine psychology (Norton, New York 1967).
17 Imperato-McMinley, J.; et al.: Androgens and the evaluation of male gender identity among male pseudo-hermaphrodites with a 5-alpha reductase deficiency. New Engl. J. Med. *300:* 1233–1237 (1979).
18 Jones, E.: The early development of female sexuality. Int. J. Psycho-Analysis *8:* 459–472 (1927).
19 Jones, J.; Samimy, J.: Plasma testosterone levels and female transsexualism. Archs sex. Behav. *2:* 251–256 (1973).
20 Kleeman, J.: The establishment of core gender identity in normal girls. I. (a) Introduction. (b) Development of the ego capacity to differentiate. Archs sex. Behav. *1:* 103–115 (1971).
21 Kleeman, J.: The establishment of core gender identity in normal girls, II. How meanings are conveyed between parent and child in the first 3 years. Archs sex. Behav. *1:* 117–129 (1971).
22 Lothstein, L.: Female-to-male transsexualism (Routledge & Kegan, London 1983).
23 Lothstein, L.: Amphetamine abuse and transsexualism. a case study. J. nerv. ment. Dis. *170:* 568–571 (1983).
24 Maccoby, E.E.: The development of sex differences (Stanford University Press, Palo Alto 1966).
25 Masters, W.: Johnson, V.: Human sexual response (Little, Brown, Boston 1966).
26 Miller, J.B.: Psychoanalysis and women (Penguin, New York 1973).
27 Money, J.; Hampson, J.; Hampson, J.: Imprinting the establishment of gender role. Archs Neurol. Psychiat. *77:* 333–336 (1975).
28 Money, J.; Ehrhardt, A.: Man and woman, boy and girl (Johns Hopkins Press, Baltimore 1972).

29 Opitz, J.; et al.: Pseudo-vaginal perineoscrotal hypospadias. Clin. Genet. *3:* 1–19 (1971).
30 Rochlin, G.: The masculine dilemma (Little, Brown, Boston 1980).
31 Roiphe, E.; Galenson, H.: Infantile origins of sexual identity (International Universities Press, New York 1981).
32 Schafer, R.: Problems in Freud's psychology of women. J. Am. psychoanal. Ass. *24:* 459–484 (1976).
33 Sendrail, M.; Gleizes, L.: Le transsexualisme féminin et la problème de ses conditions psychiques ou hormonales. Revue fr. Endocr. clin. *2:* 35–41 (1961).
34 Sherfey, M.J.: The nature and evolution of female sexuality (Vintage, New York 1966).
35 Silvers, W.; Wachtel, S.: H-Y antigen: behavior and function. Science *195:* 956–959 (1977).
36 Stoller, R.: Sex and gender (Science House, New York 1975).
37 Stoller, R.: Primary femininity. J. Am. psychoanal. Ass. *24:* 59–78 (1976).
38 Stoller, R.: A contribution to the study of gender identity: follow-up. Int. J. Psycho-Analysis *60:* 433–441 (1979).

L.M. Lothstein, PhD, Department of Psychiatry, Case Western Reserve University, University Hospitals of Cleveland, Cleveland, OH 44106 (USA)

The Psychosocial Impact of High Risk Pregnancy

Michael T. Gyves

Department of Reproductive Biology, Case Western Reserve University, University Hospitals of Cleveland, Ohio, USA

Introduction

In 1974 the American Board of Obstetrics and Gynecology officially recognized the discipline of maternal-fetal medicine as a subspeciality within the field of obstetrics. The establishment of a subspecialty for high risk obstetrics implies that there is a group of women who have or are at risk for developing complications during pregnancy and who will benefit from application of the most advanced knowledge, techniques, and technology during their pregnancies. Maternal-fetal medicine specialists (perinatologists) have as their mission, however, more than simply the care of high risk pregnant women. As a group they are also engaged in furthering our knowledge regarding normal and abnormal pregnancies and the development of newer technology to improve pregnancy outcome. Advances in the field of maternal-fetal medicine have implications for all pregnant women.

A corollary to the concept of a specialty in high risk obstetrics is that every pregnant woman can be classified as 'low risk' or 'high risk', the former being perceived as normal and the latter as 'different'. This distinction, however, is not so clear in the type of care that is afforded to the individual woman. As advances have been achieved in the field of maternal-fetal medicine, their application has spilled over from the high risk group to the low risk group of women. Whether or not this practice is appropriate is a separate and controversial issue. What is clear is that the widespread use of technology and modern techniques in obstetrical care has profound impact on many women.

Our recognition of and emphasis on high risk pregnancies has resulted in a striking reaction on the part of many consumers. They view the physicians' concern about risks as reflecting an attitude toward pregnancy as a disease state. These consumers foster pregnancy as a natural and normal event which requires little or no intervention for a good outcome. Thus there has developed among many consumers an attitude of suspicion and even mistrust toward obstetricians, who are viewed as being intrusive into a very personal event.

It is in this climate of controversy that a woman with a truly high risk pregnancy enters into the medical care system. Regardless of the philosophy of care which the obstetrician brings to the low risk pregnancy, in the high risk situation attention is focused on real or potential problems. There is an automatic tendency to treat the high risk woman as one who has an illness which warrants constant vigilance and careful intervention. Thus it becomes very clear to such a woman that she is 'different'.

High Risk Pregnancy as a Stress Factor

Any illness is an emotional stress factor and this is particularly true during pregnancy. Whereas illness is normally accompanied by fears regarding one's own immediate or future well-being, during pregnancy there is the accompanying concern about the well-being of the developing fetus. This applies more so to the woman who has experienced a prior pregnancy loss related to her high risk conditions. *Merkatz* [8] found that hospitalized high risk pregnant women exhibited at least as much anxiety and concern regarding the well-being of their babies in utero as they did for themselves. Underlying these obvious concerns there may be a serious deterioration of self-image if the individual perceives that she may not be capable of successfully completing a normal reproductive function.

For the woman who has lived with a chronic condition such as hypertension or diabetes prior to pregnancy, the focus on illness during pregnancy may be in direct contrast to a concept of health or functional normality which had been encouraged during her long-term medical care. In this way she not only comes to see herself as different from other pregnant women, but she is faced with an inner conflict between a former image of herself and a new image which is thrust upon her. Noncompliance may be the end result of this inner conflict.

Hospitalization during pregnancy enhances the fears and the emotional stresses for the high risk woman [7]. She must not only fully acknowledge the reality of her 'illness', but she must surrender her autonomy. Regression into a dependency role is a natural process for the hospitalized patient if she is to adapt to the hospital environment and routines. There is again an inner conflict between the dependency role fostered in a complicated pregnancy and the autonomy which may have been encouraged in prior years. Assumption of this 'illness' behavior may be especially difficult for the high risk woman who does not feel ill, such as the woman with diabetes or intrauterine growth retardation. Her inability to perceive her 'illness' and its implications for fetal survival may put her in direct conflict with her care givers if she cannot relinquish her autonomy.

Whether or not she can relinquish her autonomy, the woman who perceives that either she or her fetus is at risk will generally have a desire to do whatever she can to improve the chances for a good outcome. Unfortunately, although the risk may be modified, it is all too often not eliminated by the efforts of the woman and/or her obstetrician. This may lead to a sense of helplessness on the part of the patient who fears for her baby in utero but can do little or nothing on its behalf. Helplessness may potentiate the vulnerability which so often accompanies hospitalization, and may even progress to depression [11].

The Psychology of Pregnancy

Normal pregnancy is a dynamic episode of psychological development which has been variously described as 'a phase of organic growth and psychosexual development inherent in the female constitution' [1], 'a biologically determined period of psychological stress' [4], and 'a period of crisis involving profound psychological as well as somatic changes' [2]. *Bibring* [2] suggests that pregnancy is similar to adolescence and menopause in that it is a natural crisis phase which normally involves maturational change. During the process of change, the woman may exhibit behavior which, on the surface, appears regressive when compared to normal behavior in her nonpregnant state.

The psychodynamics of the psychological process of pregnancy is a complex series of adaptive steps which culminate in the attainment of a healthy mothering behavior. Successful mastery of the crisis involves working through a period of psychic disequilibrium. *Caplan* [4] describes a process in which many women initially reject the concept of pregnancy, progress through a phase of acceptance, and then recognize the reality and the identity of the fetus in preparation for motherhood. *Bibring* et al. [3] suggest two essential tasks which must be mastered in the normal maturational crisis. The first, in early pregnancy, involves a concentration on self and an integration of the fetus into this concept of self. As pregnancy progresses, particularly after quickening, the second task is undertaken. This involves recognizing the developing baby as a separate person.

According to *Rubin* [12] the pregnant woman goes through a continuum of processes in her progression toward the maternal role. In sequence, the steps of the continuum are mimicry, role play, fantasy, introjection-projection-rejection and grief work. Mimicry involves the imitation and adoption of behavioral manifestations which the woman relates to the mothering role. In role play there is an 'acting out' or 'trying on' of the mothering role. Fantasy involves imagining how the child will be, the development of a mental picture of a separate individual. In introjection-projection-rejection the woman looks to models outside of herself to provide a reinforcement of the image of herself as a mother which she is developing. Grief work is the process by which the prospective mother relinquishes her attachment to former roles or goals so that she may assume the role of mothering.

These various theories of the psychology of pregnancy involve a common theme, that of a psychological evolution. They all describe pregnancy as a dynamic process in which a woman experiences an emotional disequilibrium which must undergo a resolution for her to function well in a mothering role. That additional or unusual stresses can disrupt either the process or the ultimate equilibrium is not surprising.

Maladaptive Processes in a High Risk Pregnancy

In referring to pregnancy as a period of crisis similar to puberty and menopause, *Bibring* [2] states that such crises are 'equally the testing ground of psychological health, and we find that under unfavorable conditions they tend toward more or less severe neurotic solutions'. A high risk pregnancy often presents unfavorable conditions for the maturational process of pregnancy, and may interfere with successful attainment of the mothering role. The ease with which an individual resolves the emotional disequilibrium of pregnancy is dependent upon her own ego integration. Someone who has perceived herself as chronically ill prior to pregnancy may have insufficient ego strength to master the psychological developmental process of pregnancy. Similarly, the woman who has a past history of reproductive failures may enter pregnancy with such a poor self-image that she is unable to progress through the normal processes of maturation.

Many women have difficulty accepting pregnancy at the start [4], but the initial rejection or ambivalence usually gives way to acceptance by the end of the first trimester. On the other hand, excessive fear for her own health, or a very pessimistic view about the chances for having a live, healthy baby can interfere with the acceptance of pregnancy. Later perception of the fetus as a separate individual may also be impaired by an illness or a complication which focuses all of a woman's attention on herself and her own welfare. Extreme self-interest and concern may be appropriate for a high risk woman, but it may not permit her to look to the other person developing within her.

Not only does a pregnant woman normally recognize a separate person developing within her, but as pregnancy advances she prepares to interact with that person as her new baby. A real relationship or attachment to the fetus in utero develops from the time of quickening up to delivery so that there is already a strong bond established when a mother first sees her new baby. It is this process of attachment during the pregnancy which is most likely to be stunted during a high risk pregnancy. If a woman has a genuine fear that she will lose her baby, either before or after delivery, she does not try to establish a strong bond which must later be broken when the loss occurs. This maladaptive behavior is demonstrated vividly by a woman who has previously experienced a stillbirth or neonatal death. Her role play and fantasies during pregnancy are inhibited, and in the immediate postpartum period she tends to interact with her newborn in a mechanical way, as if she is caring for a stranger. *Bibring* [2] initially suggested that failure to complete the normal psychic maturational process by the time of delivery might lead to abnormal maternal-child interactions. This concept was later modified when *Bibring* et al. [3] concluded that maturational changes continue after delivery, and may continue as the child develops. This is borne out in the process which we see after a woman who has anticipated a loss delivers a healthy baby. The initial distant relationship gradually changes into a close bond as the mother gets to know her new baby. Attachment is not thwarted. It is simply delayed.

A history of previous pregnancy losses and fear of another loss may sometimes lead to a pathological relationship between parents and child, referred to as the 'vulnerable child syndrome' [6]. These parents become overly protective, overly concerned and unable to discipline the child. The child in such a relationship often suffers with abnormal psychosocial development.

Problems which interfere with the normal adaptive processes in pregnancy certainly put the mother-child relationship in jeopardy. They also put the mother's overall emotional health in continuing jeopardy. A woman who is psychologically ill prepared for the mothering role may be devastated when this role is inevitably thrust upon her at parturition. *Cohen* [5] believes that postpartum psychoses may often have their origins in failure to complete the normal adaptive processes of pregnancy. Knowing who is at risk for such serious sequelae, we may be able to improve long-term outcomes with close attention to and early intervention for the woman in need.

The Family

The family figures prominently in the stresses which occur in a high risk pregnancy. Admission of a pregnant woman to the hospital precipitates stress within the family, and this increases the stress which the patient herself experiences. In her study of hospitalized high risk women, *Merkatz* [8] noted that worry about husband and children at home ranked high on a list of concerns. She found more distress among hospitalized pregnant women who had children at home than among those who did not have dependent children. The highest stress ratings in her entire study group were recorded for women who had children at home. Family members may also increase stress and conflicts for the hospitalized high risk woman if they fail to perceive that she truly has an illness or a risk to the fetus. This results in a lack of emotional support from the family, and a greater sense of vulnerability on the part of the patient.

Caplan [4] states that during pregnancy a woman exhibits 'increased introversion and dependency', accompanied by 'increased demands for nurturance'. The husband, who would normally be perfectly willing and able to provide the support and affection required, might find it difficult to do so if he is faced with a high risk situation. If the fetus is at risk, he may be distracted from his wife's needs by an excessive concern for the baby-to-be, or he may even feel resentful toward her because her illness jeopardizes his child. On the other hand, if the woman's health is threatened, her spouse may be beset by guilt feelings because he put her at risk by impregnating her. Such feelings may be accompanied by a sense of inadequacy when he realizes that he is unable to alter her status by any intervention on his part. The support role may not survive resentment, guilt, and inadequacy.

The simple process of hospital admission also interferes with the nurturing role of the spouse. Whereas the husband was at one time an integral part of the pregnancy experience, he abruptly finds himself to be an outsider, physically separated from his wife for all but a few hours of visiting each day.

Some families adapt very well to the problems of a high risk pregnancy. The husband may rise to the occasion, providing all possible support for his hospitalized or bedridden wife while, at the same time, being father and mother for the other children at home. He may have such concern for his wife's welfare, that he not only provides her with nurturance, but also with smothering protection. This adaptation to new roles may work well until the woman herself has delivered, recovered, and returned home to assume her own mothering role. A conflict may then develop if the spouse cannot relinquish his protector role and permit his wife to grow out of her dependency.

We can see then that high risk pregnancy brings many stresses to bear on families. With resentment, guilt, lack of emotional support, overprotective behavior, and role conflicts, it is not surprising that many marriages suffer severe setbacks and even disintegrate because of pregnancy complications.

Emotional Benefits of High Risk Care

Although both a high risk condition and the special interventions which are necessitated by that condition may be sources of stress during pregnancy, it should not be presumed that intensive perinatal care itself inevitably produces emotional stress for the high risk patient. In fact, modern obstetrical care may actually reduce the anxiety experienced by many high risk patients and their spouses.

Appropriate reassurance must be a constant theme in the care of women at risk, and some diagnostic techniques provide more reassurance than the most supportive statement from a physician. Couples who are at high risk for bearing a child with a genetic or chromosomal abnormality will be under great stress until they know that the risk is not realized. Prenatal diagnostic studies, i.e., amniocentesis and ultrasound, can provide the couple with valuable information early in the pregnancy. If the findings are normal, they may be spared many months of anxious waiting.

The intermittent use of ultrasound as pregnancy progresses may provide continued reassurance concerning fetal well-being when the fetus is at risk. An additional benefit of ultrasound examination is that it accelerates the recognition and acceptance by the woman of the reality and separate identity of her fetus. As mentioned earlier, when loss of the fetus or newborn is a real fear, attachment may be delayed. Real-time ultrasound imaging of the fetus in utero may accelerate attachment [9], and so counterbalance some of the emotional debt which the fear of loss incurs.

Hospitalization has already been cited as a significant stress factor, but it may sometimes reduce stress. The woman who has previously experienced a loss may derive great relief of anxiety from being in the hospital [8]. Attentiveness by the staff plus the close fetal surveillance provided with antepartum electronic fetal monitoring and biochemical testing of fetal well-being can provide considerable reassurance.

Widespread use of continuous electronic fetal monitoring in labor is still a controversial issue, with objections coming from those low risk couples who view it as an unnecessary intrusion. The vast majority of high risk couples, however, look positively upon continuous fetal monitoring in labor [10, 13, 14]. For them it is a security blanket which provides a continuous status report on the fetus.

It should be clear then that for many high risk couples intensive perinatal care provides both an objective and a subjective benefit.

The Care Givers

There is considerable interest in the psychological impact of a high risk pregnancy and intensive perinatal care upon the pregnant woman and her family. But what about her care givers? They are subject to emotional stresses in all phases of perinatal care.

A stressful situation arises for the obstetrician with the first suspicion of a complication during pregnancy. In part this relates to the lack of precision of our diagnostic tools, such that it is often difficult to differentiate between the extremes of normal and the midly abnormal. If there is any uncertainly about whether or not a problem is developing, the physician is faced with a dilemma. Revealing to the patient that there may be a problem will precipitate anxiety on her part. On the other hand, waiting for more definitive data may spare unnecessary patient anxiety, but it burdens the physician with the responsibility for any disaster which might result from failure to intervene in a timely fashion.

When problems are unequivocal, solutions may not be so clear. Many controversies exist regarding the 'best' course of action to take in a variety of high risk situations. If the appropriate intervention is controversial, options must be discussed with the patient and her husband. They may choose an option which differs from that preferred by the care givers, thus precipitating more stress for the medical care team.

Even when the appropriate course of action cannot be disputed, the perinatal team carries a heavy load of responsibility. They are sometimes imbued with superhuman qualities by the patient and her family who presume that a perfect outcome is assured regardless of the antecedent complications. Being equated with deities leaves no room for error and imposes a unique kind of stress.

With the best of care, a happy outcome for a high risk pregnancy is not always realized. The practice of maternal-fetal medicine may be likened to a roller coaster ride of emotions, a series of highs and lows. One day the staff may share exhilirating joy with new parents whom they have helped through a precarious pregnancy. The next day they may be facilitating the grief work of a couple who have suffered an inevitable but tragic loss. As rewarding as all of this work is, it carries with it a real risk of emotional exhaustion. We must be mindful, therefore, not only to provide support for our patients who are experiencing emotional stress, but also to be alert for and attentive to the emotional needs of ourselves and our colleagues.

References

1 Benedek, T.: Psychobiological aspects of mothering. Am. J. Orthopsychiat. *26:* 272–278 (1956).
2 Bibring, G.L.: Some considerations of the psychological processes in pregnancy. Psychoanal. Study Child *14:* 113–121 (1959).
3 Bibring, G.L.; Dwyer, T.F.; Huntington, D.S.; Valenstein, A.F.: A study of the psychological processes in pregnancy and of the earliest mother-child relationship. I. Some propositions and comments. Psychoanal. Study Child *16:* 9–72 (1961).
4 Caplan, G.: Emotional implications of pregnancy and influences on family relationships; in Stuart, Prugh, The healthy child, pp. 72–81 (Harvard University Press, Cambridge 1960).
5 Cohen, R.L.: Some maladaptive syndromes of pregnancy and puerperium. Obstet. Gynec., N.Y. *27:* 562–570 (1966).

6 Green, M.; Solnit, A.J.: Reactions to the threatened loss of a child: a vulnerable child syndrome. Pediatrics, Springfield *34:* 58–66 (1964).
7 Lucente, F.E.; Fleck, S.: A study of hospitalization anxiety in 408 medical and surgical patients. Psychosom. Med. *34:* 304–312 (1972).
8 Merkatz, R.B.: Behavior of hospitalized high risk maternity patients; Masters thesis Case Western Reserve University, Frances Payne Bolton School of Nursing (1976) (unpublished).
9 Milne, L.S.; Rich, O.J.: Cognitive and affective aspects of the responses of pregnant women to sonography. Mat.-Child Nurs. J. *10:* 15–40 (1981).
10 Molfese, V.; Sunshine, P.; Bennett, A.: Reactions of women to intrapartum fetal monitoring. Obstet. Gynec., N.Y. *59:* 705–709 (1982).
11 Penticuff, J.H.: Psychologic implications in high-risk pregnancy. Nurs. Clin. N. Am. *17:* 69–78 (1982).
12 Rubin, R.: Attainment of the maternal role. Part I. Processes. Nurs. Res. *16:* 237–245 (1967).
13 Shields, D.: Maternal reactions to fetal monitoring. Am. J. Nurs. *78:* 2110–2112 (1978).
14 Starkman, M.N.: Fetal monitoring: psychologic consequences and management recommendations. Obstet. Gynec., N.Y. *50:* 500–504 (1977).

Michael T. Gyves, MD, Director, Department of Obstetrics and Gynecology, Saint Luke's Hospital, 11311 Shaker Boulevard, Cleveland, Ohio 44104

A Modest Proposal: Breastfeeding for the Infants of Adolescent Mothers

Nada L. Stotland[a], Christine Peterson[b]

[a]Department of Psychiatry, Pritzker School of Medicine, University of Chicago, and Psychiatric Liasion to Obstetrics and Gynecology, Michael Reese Hospital, Chicago, Ill.; [b]Department of Obstetrics and Gynecology, Georgetown University School of Medicine, Washington, D.C., USA

Adolescent mothers in the United States do not breast-feed their infants. When we, a psychiatrist and an obstetrician, made this observation, we discovered that this situation was well known to the staffs at major medical centers. Indeed it was taken for granted and it was rationalized. Beyond the occasional poster, pamphlet, or hospital feeding class no attention or effort was directed at it. In fact, literature review revealed that the finding was neither documented nor understood [7]. Few, if any, studies of feeding practices even offered mother's age as a variable [1].

This informational lacuna existed and continues to exist, in a sea of studies and data about two intimately related issues; teenage pregnancy and infant feeding. Teenage pregnancy, is considered to be a problem of epidemic proportions [9]. Despite intense attention in the popular press and numerous studies [13], aimed at prevention, there has been no major impact on the statistics [12]. Neither the national government strategy of promoting chastity nor the economic and psychological vicious cycle of inner city life offer any immediate promise of change. And relatively little attention has been paid to the postpartum teenager, her parenting, and her child. A classic study followed a cohort of all the first graders in a slum neighborhood for 15 years and identified some high-risk factors, notably the household consisting only of mother and children. Risk of poor outcome also takes a significant jump when the family increases from 1 to 2 or more children per adolescent mother.

There is some disagreement about the maternal performance of adolescents. For one thing, this is quite a heterogeneous group. One might expect a wide gap in maternal maturity – empathy, tolerance for frustration, ability to postpone gratification, realistic expectation of infants –

between a single 13-year-old eighth grader and a married 19-year-old [17].

There may also be a significant difference in physiologic readiness, as reflected in complications of pregnancy and delivery. Here again there is disagreement in the literature. Although the existing figures indicate greater morbidity in the younger population, it is not clear whether this is secondary to age per se or to concomitant conditions such as poor nutrition and inadequate prenatal care in the younger mothers. A study at the University of Michigan some years ago indicated that nutritional supplementation and good obstetric care led to equivalent obstetric outcomes in lower class adolescent and middle class older mothers. The most recent data indicate that while other risks even out with intense support, an increased rate of prematurity persists in the adolescent population.

In any case, as it now stands, the young mother and her infant are at high risk in our society. They are overrepresented in populations of prematures, hospital admissions, and perinatal mortality. It is often said that the inner city of Chicago has perinatal mortality comparable to Third World countries. Many groups are attempting constructive interventions with mother-infant dyads observed or predicted to be malfunctioning. *Fraiberg* [3] described her work with such a population in a paper in *Adolescent Psychiatry*. Although some of these programs pick up subjects referred prenatally, many admit only those identified weeks – or more often months – after delivery [15]. Some programs offer support to a small cross-section, such as a school or clinic, but most address only the population thought to be at maximum risk. The vast majority of adolescent mother/infant dyads are begrudged minimal economic support, perhaps some nutritional supplementation, and otherwise left to fend for themselves as well as they can.

The second relevant area is infant feeding. A good deal is known about its physiology, history, and sociology. While breast-feeding by the mother is the method which has sustained the human race through the vast majority of its history, attempts at artificial feeding have been documented since hundreds of years before the birth of Christ. Various flour, bread, sugar and water 'pap' were concocted, with animal milks used less frequently. Well-to-do mothers in ancient Greece and Rome resorted instead to carefully chosen wet nurses to free them for other pastimes while insuring proven nutritional sources for their babies. Infants in the 17th and 18th century French aristocracy were less fortunate. Large numbers of them were farmed out to be boarded in the countryside. There were almost no children among the thousands of people at Versailles, for example. Wet nurses often saw to several children at once and the mortality rate [4] was over 50%. Until the 1940s, however, maternal breast-feeding was the modal behavior all over the world. Astute pediatricians published many studies documenting lower rates of mortality and respiratory [20, 22] and digestive morbidity in breast-fed as compared with artificially fed infants.

In the 1930s, 40s, and 50s, natural functions came to be looked upon as less clean, scientific, controllable, modern, and civilized than technical ones. Birth moved from home to hospital and was managed via analgesia, anesthesia, and instrumentation. Feedings were mixed, measured, sterilized, and timed. Mothers who nursed were openly referred to as animal throwbacks. All of these 'advances' began in the upper socioeconomic classes and gravitated downwards, connoting, like contraception, sophistication, freedom from bodily imperatives, and a curious combination of sexiness and prudery. By the early 60s, breast-feeding in the USA was at an all-time low. The spread to the underdeveloped countries, vigorously encouraged by the formula companies, sparked concern and finally a major collaborative 9-country study by the World Health Organization [6] aimed at understanding and then reversing it.

The reasons for this concern are not all confined to the Third World and, in fact, are quite pertinent to (our) inner-city adolescent mothers. Their infants are at increased risk of serious morbidity and mortality from infectious diseases, failure to thrive, neglect, abuse, and adolescent parenthood. In Chicago, fewer than half of the mothers finish high school and become employed or employable [9]. Often their lack of parenting skills and their deficient circumstances prevent the realization of their fantasies in a gratifying parenthood.

Mother's milk is still the optimum infant nutrition. Breast-fed infants have significantly fewer digestive disturbances, gastrointestinal and other major infections, and allergies, and increased immunity to a number of illnesses [2]. Even in Third World populations much more severely nutritionally deprived than our inner city, the mother's breast milk decreases in quantity, rather than quality [23]. It cannot be diluted with unclean – or too much – water, over- or underheated. Kept in its natural container, it cannot spoil or run out during a day's outing or between welfare checks. Cow's milk has too much protein and forms larger, less digestible curds in the stomach. Comparative studies on milk of various mammalian species strongly suggest that the natural feeding style of the human infants is most likely that of creatures which are kept near the mother and nurse on and off at will or at 1- to 2-hour intervals at most [21]. (This news comes as a relief to young upper middle class mothers, the first generation to return to nursing babies, whose mothers and husbands frequently complain that the baby is 'at it again'!) [10]. This provides for a great deal of mother-infant contact [19]. The breast cannot be propped in the crib. The American Academy of Pediatrics Committee on Nutrition [Dr. *Lockhart,* pers. commun.] has taken the position that an adolescent capable of conception is physiologically capable of pregnancy, delivery, and lactation if given adequate nutritional intake. They issued first a statement unequivocally advocating breast-feeding over artificial feeding and then a statement underscoring the responsibility of health care professionals to promote and support it.

How are we doing so far? We began by noting (1) adolescents do not breast-feed, and (2) we are doing so little about it that we don't even know it. In the final stages of preparing the draft of this paper, we tried to get the latest figure from our own large institution. Although we have computerized peripartum data, the only piece of feeding information elicited is the prospective mother's professed intent when she is admitted in labor. We reasoned that this would probably correlate highly if not perfectly with her immediate postpartum behavior. However, these data are not now accessible in the monthly statistics. They will remain in the computer until a special program is written to retrieve them. There is no other centralized record kept. In the course of this search, we did learn from the nurse clinician who examines a good proportion of the babies that, 'I have had 3 adolescent mothers breast-feed babies in the 7 years I have been here'.

Our knowledge gap and laissez-faire attitude are not congruent with our attention to other procedures and patient behaviors which have much less proven merit. One problem is the assumption that for this population, breast-feeding would be impossible or even inadvisable to achieve. There are some significant issues to consider. The first is the current state of intervention. Most major university hospitals have some sort of classes and printed material about breast-feeding available both in the prenatal clinic and during the patient's ever briefer stay on the postpartum floors. A typical educational poster supplied by the International Childbirth Education Association is a line drawing of a mother gazing lovingly at the infant at one breast. She is nude to the waist. For educational purposes, the milk ducts and lobules of her second breast have been drawn in anatomically. There is good reason to suspect that does not address the psychological needs of the pregnant inner-city adolescent.

The paucity of suitable educational material is merely an external manifestation of the defeatist attitudes of hospital staffs towards this situation. These kinds of situations tend to become vicious cycles – or self-fulfilling prophecies. However, when one of us was a pediatric intern, in 1968, a prominent attending obstetrician insisted that upper middle class fathers could never be allowed in delivery rooms because their wives would always demand so much sedation in labor that their babies would have to be vigorously resuscitated at birth. Only a few years later such a father-to-be and obstetrician from this same hospital went to court to insist on his right to be present at birth, and nowadays it is 'de rigeur'. Similarly, a lactation support team working hospitals in the New York City ghetto seems to be responsible for dramatic changes in the incidence of breast-feeding in a population similar to ours. Age-specific rates, again, are not yet available. There are early successful returns from other pilot programs around the country as well [5].

This brings us to the second issue, that of current cultural and familial infant feeding patterns and support systems for adolescents [16]. Breast-feeding is correlated at this point in time with high socioeconomic status [18], though in the inner city it may seem a throwback to the southern sharecrop farm. It can be argued, on the basis of a variety of studies, that a mother's selection of infant feeding method is dependent on the attitude of the baby's father, the health care providers, or her own mother, as reflected in current statements and behaviors and in how she fed the subject in subject's infancy [2]. We might expect the effects of mothers to be increased by the fact that adolescents are more likely to live with and depend physically and psychologically on their mothers than older pregnant women [8]. Teenagers are encouraged to return to and finish school and prepare for a financially self-supporting life. It is assumed that artificial feeding is the only form consistent with that aim. However, follow-up studies indicate that a minority of adolescent mothers return to school and even fewer graduate. Their mothers' role in caring for the grandchild falls off rapidly over time, leaving the adolescent most often with virtually all the psychological and physical responsibility for parenting. While the advantages of education and work are clear, the possibility of their attainment is both questionable and postponable. Meanwhile the baby is here now and real. A highly sensitive, probably crucial, period in its development is proceeding physiologically and psychologically. What internal resources does the adolescent mother bring to meet her infants' needs? The effects her maternal functioning has on her child can be expected to make a significant impact on the adolescent mother's comfort, continuing ability to function, and self-esteem.

A great deal has been written about the development of normal and deviant adolescents [11]. Adolescent pregnancy as a social concern engendered a spate of studies on adolescents attitudes, behaviors, and reactions in the areas of sexuality, contraception, and abortion [16]. Very little has been published about the adolescent as a mother or even soon-to-be mother. It is a painful subject to study. We will attempt to identify some issues in adolescent development which bear on parenting and specifically on infant feeding.

Hatcher's [14] 1973 paper on 'The Adolescent Experience of Pregnancy and Abortion' takes a developmental perspective. Although *Hatcher's* subjects were white, middle-class abortion applicants, that orientation is conceptually useful, as is her schema of the issues involved. It is important to remember both that an enormous amount of development and change highly relevant to parenting potential occurs during the course of adolescence, and that the stage of development may or may not be congruent with chronological age.

She first summarizes some major areas of development as they are expressed in the progress through adolescence in general. Secondly she identifies eight variables specifically related to pregnancy and describes the findings in each area in subjects already classified in the first scheme as early, middle, or late adolescents. Our research subjects fall chronologically into the middle segment. We made no independent developmental assessments. Presumably they covered the whole range. We can readily point out high points relative both to adolescents' attitudes towards breast-feeding and to implications for intervention. The pregnant early adolescent has little accurate reproductive knowledge, but some interest in testing out new bodily functions and in rebelling against her mother. She has trouble facing the reality of the pregnancy, the fetus, or herself as a mother, sees things in black and white, and feels helpless about the future. The middle adolescent is more oedipal, with more knowledge, more sense of her own femininity and pregnancy and some beginning notion of motherhood and babies. She is ambivalent about the future. Attempts to grapple with the breast-feeding issue must focus, then, on relationships with significant others, cognitive knowledge, motivations for pregnancy, and the ability to cognitively and emotionally handle the realities of motherhood.

Discussion

An interesting and compelling question arises. What are the sequelae of being in a situation for which one is developmentally unprepared? A person may regress, become fixated, or grow. Although adolescent motherhood presents some severe difficulties in our society, in other places in time and space it has been, complete with breast-feeding, the mode. Again, breast-feeding might represent an additional and overwhelming demand on the organism, or, alternatively, a means of achieving and demonstrating mastery in life's most challenging (and important) role. Intervention studies of various populations of mothers with deficient maternal skills and presumably poor psychological resources have revealed that support and modeling of desirable behaviors can lead to clinically significant changes in feelings, skills, and outcomes. Although it would require sensitivity to the multi-layered issues involved, knowledgeable and emphatic support of adolescent breast-feeding might result in not only healthier infants, but also more gratified mothers. It is not unreasonable, even, to hypothesize that successful mothering might be as much of a spur to effective future family planning as contraceptive availability, economic constraints, and sermons on chastity.

Conclusions

In our society at present, we have singled out adolescent motherhood as an important issue, albeit one to which we give more expressed concern than constructive attention. Perhaps a combination of denial, rage, and frustration results in our failure to offer more than token and sporadic support to this presumably stressed mother-child population. Perhaps it seems that hoping to elicit maternal behavior from a child is like expecting a turnip to yield blood, an exercise in futility. However, we have no alternative blood bank. One of the resources these mothers demonstrably possess is their physiologic nursing capacity – their milk. Perhaps it is a disservice to all concerned that caregivers have given up the hope of tapping it without exploring the pros and cons in any depth. Some studies indicate that interventions can change feeding behavior in a previously poorly informed and served population. We have attempted to open the subject for consideration in the adolescent population. Until we have attempted to respond with specialized educational materials and programs geared to their social situations and psychological dynamics, it is a dereliction of duty to conclude that this state of affairs is either undesirable or impossible to address.

Epilogue

Lest the reader assume that our investment in this issue begins with background information and ends with exhortation, we will briefly describe our study, 'Adolescents' Attitudes toward Breast-feeding', already well underway. We have conducted structured interviews with pregnant and non-pregnant adolescent girls. Information gathered begins with demographic and socioeconomic variables. Next we address aspects of knowledge about infant care and feeding, with particular attention to information about bottle and breast-feeding. We ask what experiences, attitudes, information, and suggestions have been offered, and by whom ot what. We want to know who usually has the most impact on the girl's behavior, how and with whom she spends her time, and what are her plans for life and infant feeding postpartum (in the future for the nonpregnant population). Lastly we ask the subject's opinion regarding her ability to breast-feed, and the advantages and disadvantages for the mother.

Preliminary results confirm our hypothesis that interest in, knowledge of, and plans for breast-feeding are correlated with higher socioeconomic – and nonpregnant – status.

The very persons for whom valid and positive breast-feeding information is most important are either not being given this information, or perhaps, are not perceiving the information given as valid or positive in any way that has meaning for them!

It can be postulated that pregnancy is either the cause *or* the result of the same personal and environmental factors that lead to the different perceptions of breast-feeding information. In other words, the fact of being pregnant *itself* may pressure the adolescent into failing to acknowledge some of the information she is presented with. The pregnant adolescent invariably is barraged by a large amount of directive advice, often with contradictory and conflicting content. In an effort to cope with her situation and to make decisions in this context, she may need to deny ever having received portions of this information or advice. She may make decisions based not on the content of the information given, but on the emotional significance to her of the individual or circumstances from which she receives the information.

On the other hand, the material, social, and emotional deprivations which often set the stage for adolescent pregnancy may also provide an inhospitable situation for receipt and processing of information about an activity which is going to require that the adolescent *give* to another human being the attention, warmth, and bodily intimacy she so craves for herself. She may have gotten pregnant in her search for caring attention, and may not be able to, so intimately and directly, give to her infant what she never received herself. The interposition of an inanimate object between herself and her baby may ease the feeling of seeing her own unmet dependency needs mirrored in her infant.

When statistical analyses and conceptual considerations are complete, results cannot only be shared, but also serve as the basis for a pilot intervention program. We hope that the present paper will encourage other investigators and caregivers to involve themselves with this interesting, important, and poorly understood issue.

Acknowledgements

Thanks to: *Monica Schwartz, Carol Ballou, Barbara Cramer, Lea Stotland, Young-Ran Chung, Ilene Lanin-Kettering, Martin Harrow, Mary Rogel.*

References

1 Contemporary patterns of breast-feeding. Report on the WHO Collaborative Study on Breast-Feeding (WHO, Geneva 1981).
2 Lawrence, R.A.: Breast-feeding. A guide for the medical profession (Mosby, St. Louis 1980).
3 Fraiberg, S.: The adolescent mother and her infant; in: Adolescent psychiatry (University of Chicago, Chicago 1982).
4 Lloyd de Mause (ed.): The history of childhood (Psychohistory Press, New York 1973).
5 Lewis, L.: Successful breast feeding programs for low-income minority mothers. Publ. Hlth Curr. (Ross Laboratories, Columbus 1982).
6 Bergevin, Y.; et al.: Do infant formula samples shorten the duration of breast-feeding? Lancet *i:* 1148 (1983).
7 National Institute of Child Health and Human Development: Selected bibliography on human milk and breast-feeding, April 7, 1983.
8 Berzonsky, M.D. (ed.): Adolescent development (Macmillan, New York 1981).
9 Teenage pregnancy. We're doing something about it. Illinois Caucus on Teenage Pregnancy.

10 Peters, D.C.; Worthington-Roberts, B.: Infant feeding practices of middle-class breast-feeding and formula-feeding mothers. Birth 9/2 (1982).
11 Offer, D.: The self-image of normal adolescents: 1962–1982; in Clinical update in adolescent psychiatry, vol. 1, No. 5 (Nassau Publications, Princeton 1983).
12 Teenagers and family planning: the need for preventive services. Fact sheet (Planned Parenthood Federation of America, New York 1981).
13 Zuehlke, M.E.: Current issues in adolescent contraceptive use. Symposium paper presented at Annual Illinois Psychiatric Society Meeting, Rosemont, Illinois (1983).
14 Hatcher, S.L.M.: The adolescent experience of pregnancy and abortion: a developmental analysis. J. Youth Adolescence 2/1 (1973).
15 Breast-feeding. Department of Human Services Commission of Public Health DC. WIC Program and the Bureau of Maternal and Child Health, Washington, DC.
16 Barglow, P.; Weinstein, S.: Therapeutic abortion during adolescence: psychiatric oberservations. J. Youth Adolescence 2/4 (1973).
17 Berg, P.W.P.; Bornstein, M.; Exum, D.B.; et al.: Some psychiatric aspects of illegitimate pregnancy in early adolescence. 1967 Annu. Meet. Am. Orthopsychiat. Ass. Washington, DC/Crittenton Comprehensive Care Center, Chicago 1967.
18 Cole, J.P.: Table 1–4. Mother's education and projected feeding choice. Clin. Pediat. 16: 352 (1977).
19 Klaus, M.H.; Kennel, J.H.: Maternal-infant bonding, the impact of early separation or loss on family development (Mosby, St. Louis 1976).
20 Langstein, R.: Value of natural feeding. Atlas der Hygiene des Säuglings und Kleinkindes (Springer, Berlin 1918).
21 Lozoff, B.; et al.: Table 8–5. J. Pediat. 91: 1 (1977).
22 Hanafy, M.M.; et al.: Table 9–4. J. Trop. Pediat. 18: 188 (1972).
23 Worthington, B.S.; Vermeersch, J.; and Williams, S.R. (eds.): Nutrition in pregnancy and lactation (Mosby, St. Louis 1977).

N.L. Stotland, MD, Pritzker School of Medicine, University of Chicago,
Psychiatric Liaison to Obstetrics and Gynecology, Michael Reese Hospital,
Chicago, IL 60616 (USA)

Psychological Implications of Recent Developments in Peripartum Care[1]

Nada L. Stotland

Psychiatric Liaison to Obstetrics and Gynecology, Michael Reese Hospital, and University of Chicago, Pritzker School of Medicine, Chicago, Ill., USA

The last 15–20 years have seen significant changes in the approach of the American middle and upper classes to childbirth [7]. In this group 40 or so years ago, the responsibility of the parent-to-be began 2 or 3 months after conception. It consisted of locating a physician who delivered babies and following his advice. There were a few educational pamphlets, books and classes for the curious, but generally they concluded as the encounter with the obstetrician began with the suggestion to 'leave it to the doctor'. The doctor generally advised strict limitations on weight gain, a salt-restricted and milk-intensive diet and a number of intercourse-free months at prescribed stages. 'Supportive' garments for the pregnant breasts, abdomen and legs were often prescribed. Vigorous activity was thought to be dangerous. Most women who had outside jobs stopped working well before delivery and stayed home until children reached school age or left home. Delivery itself was accomplished via an array of drugs including sedatives, amnestics, analgesics, tranquilizers and general anesthetics and techniques including full shaving of public hair, enema, episiotomy, outlet forceps and practices including mandatory supine and lithotomy positions, prohibition of oral intake, transfer from labor to delivery room and banning of friends and relatives from the latter and sometimes the former. Hospital stays were a week or more with the length of the stay a mark of the prestige of the attending physician. A considerable proportion of the hospital postpartum stay was spent at bed rest. All of these rituals were either taken for granted or lauded as great advancements in obstetric care. Few controlled studies

---

[1] Based upon a presentation at the American Society for Psychosomatic Obstetrics and Gynecology Meetings, Sarasota, 1984.

were performed to document their salutary medical effect and little question was raised about their psychological effects.

Concurrent falls in maternal and infant mortality seemed proof enough. Prolonged sedation and debilitation of mother and child, which were likely secondary to anesthetics and bed rest, were ascribed to childbirth itself and reinforced the feeling that the helpless parturient needed authoritarian guidance, care and intervention [8]. The social and medical approaches to childbirth in 1984 offer, in some respects, a dramatic contrast and in others 'plus ça change, plus c'est la même chose'. With a vast new array of diagnostic and therapeutic modalities and quantum leaps in consumer sophistication and expectations, prospective parents [12] face a bewildering and ofttimes conflicting array of choices, responsibilities and demands. The birth of a child is a central event in its life and that of its parents. The experience has profound and far-reaching psychological implications. And there are reasons to believe that that experience is different today than at any time in the past. This paper is intended as an overview to acquaint mental health professionals with recent developments in obstetrics, pediatrics and genetics and to help practitioners in the latter fields focus their attention on the psychiatric aspect of their work. Very few, if any, formal studies of these issues have been completed, although some are contemplated and even begun. At this point of few answers, we can and must raise many questions.

The mother of one of my colleagues complained paradoxically to her several years ago about the effect of contraception on her life. She said, 'For my mother, having children was God's will. As each one came along she did the best she could to raise it properly. For me, having children is an individual choice so I feel obligated to provide the best of everything.' This anecdote crystalizes some of the issues for people of childbearing age today. It illustrates a concern beginning before conception. Perhaps this sort of concern can be traced back to ancient fears about the sins of the fathers being visited upon the children. Certainly this psychological dynamic still holds in many cases. For the moment I would like to proceed through the reproductive cycle, more or less chronologically, in order to describe obstetrical and other developments which have taken place at each stage. This will provide a basis for the discussion of the psychological demands, advantages, disadvantages, and treatment implications of the new behaviors and methodology.

When contemplating childbearing, people today have three groups of relatively new options. They may choose to have chromosomal or genetic studies performed to determine if they are carriers of conditions medically significant to their offspring. They may learn, for example, whether they are potentially parents of a child with sickle cell anemia, or Tay-Sachs disease. First they must be aware that these tests are available. They must overcome disinclination and denial in making the decision to have the test performed and then if the results are positive, they must take them into account when making decisions about marriage and parenthood. Serum antibody levels can also be performed to determine whether a woman is susceptible to or was previously infected with illnesses, such as rubella and toxoplasmosis, with reproductive consequences.

The next group of issues come up for all potential parents. Recently published studies have raised questions about the validity of formerly used guidelines for the optimal age of childbearing. Although some caveats and risks remain, it would seem that the relatively young, that is to say, 16- to 20-, and relatively old, that is to say 35- to 45-year-old women may bear children with safety and outcome comparable to, if not quite equal to, women between 20 and 35. Though fertility decreases considerably in the older age-group and though obstetricians may still advise for that and other reasons that their patients choose to confine their childbearing to the years between 25 and 35, the biological imperatives are less compelling. Thus, there is more room for the consideration of complexities, such as career pathway, life-style, psychological readiness and physical energy. Thirdly, in the event that expected or wished for pregnancy does not occur, infertility is no longer a cause for resignation. At the outset, the medical system will intrude itself into the bedroom at the request of the couple complaining of infertility, with a vast array of basal temperature charts, timed intercourse and postcoital samplings. Reproductive endocrinology, as a recognized subspecialty, can offer a vast array of hormonal, radiographic and operative techniques for assessment and treatment [*J. Boster:* High tech. reproduction, pers. commun.]. The boundaries of the curable are constantly expanding. Microsurgical techniques have been extremely successful in restoring patency of reproductive structures in both male and female, and thereby helping a large proportion of previously hopelessly infertile men and women to achieve pregnancy [1]. In vitro fertilization is only the most expensive, visible example in a vast array of costly and exhausting, but horizon-widening technology. Even if all these techniques fail or do not apply to a particular individual, there are other possibilities besides adoption or resignation to consider. Artificial insemination is increasingly popular and has come to be employed not only by obstetricians caring for married couples, but also for single women and in free-standing self-help facilities. The flash-frozen semen of Nobel prize winners is available through an independently funded foundation and the resultant offspring and their mothers are featured on the covers of national magazines. In the case of female infertility it is the so-called surrogate mothers who are featured on national magazines, wearing tee shirts with arrows pointing to their pregnant bellies and legends 'this space for hire'. Despite some biblical references, this discongruity between the biological and legal family is a relatively new social phenomenon [5].

Once the pregnancy has been decided upon and achieved, another whole array of possibilities impends. There is immediately the decision whether to carry the pregnancy to term or to have an elective abortion based on personal needs and resources. Then, within weeks of conception, a variety of tests can be performed in an effort to determine the baby's genetic and physical condition [12]. For some years amniocentesis has been recommended for those over a given age, approximately 35, and for those at known genetic risk. The physical risk of the procedure itself are in some dispute, but most likely quite small. The results of the amniocentesis are not available until the second trimester of pregnancy. Then, there is some dispute about the advisability of the procedure for anyone who does not plan to have a second trimester abortion in the event of an adverse diagnosis. Chorionic villi sampling can be performed earler in pregnancy and offers an immediate, that is to say, 1- to 2-day, diagnosis. An abortion, if decided upon, can be performed in the first trimester. However, the main advantage described by the geneticist involved in the pioneer program of this procedure at Michael Reese Hospital in Chicago was the preservation of the family's privacy. The whole process can easily be completed before anyone besides the parents and treatment team are aware of the pregnancy.

Blood tests of the mother for alpha-fetal protein can enable the physician to make a diagnosis of neurotube defects in the unborn child. At the time of this writing this test has been determined to be not cost effective for the American population since these defects are less common here than in other countries, notably Great Britain. However, the test can be elected by an individual and her physician if the appropriate laboratory facilities are available [15].

The next procedure most pregnant women will encounter is the ultrasound examination of the pregnant uterus. This test is an early routine, at least in major medical centers and urban private practices. Recent studies indicate that an accurate diagnosis of fetal sex can be made by ultrasound examination in the second trimester of pregnancy, thereby raising the questions, as has amniocentesis for some time, of the psychological and moral implications of the availability of this knowledge to parents before birth [16]. At this point in time, however, the determination of sex is an incidental one in ultrasound use in pregnancy. Serial ultrasound enables the obstetric team to more accurately date the pregnancy, prognosticate about the date of delivery and to identify clinically significant medical conditions. Here is a recent case example:

A healthy, happily married 30-year-old woman presented for obstetric care of her first pregnancy. In the course of routine serial ultrasound examination the fetus was noted to have a renal abnormality. In the opinion of the perinatologist this abnormality would require surgical intervention 1–2 days after birth. The mother had planned to deliver at a very fine woman's hospital in a large metropolitan area. The hospital was equipped with a neonatal intensive care unit, but was not equipped for neonatal surgery. The baby, if born in this hospital, would have to be transferred to another children's unit for care. Estimates of fetal size and position were such that a cesarean section was a strong possibility. Therefore, it was unlikely that the mother would be able comfortably to have contact with her newborn for some days after delivery if it were not in the same hospital where she delivered. By virtue of a great deal of careful thought and legwork, a plan was arranged whereby the mother's familiar, trusted and highly competent obstetrician would induce labor at a prearranged time and deliver her at another hospital, where care for both her and the baby was available. In this case a major conflict of interest seems to have been avoided. However, the practice of prenatal exchange transfusion and prenatal fetal surgery raises new issues somewhat conceptually related to the bodily integrity issue in abortion and to the debates which I remember from my medical school days in the 60s about whether a mother's or baby's life should be saved in the event of an obstetrical catastrophe. In actuality, very few, if any, of these situations ever arose. The need for fetal surgery will likewise probably remain rare, but it has attracted a good deal of popular attention, as exemplified by a cover article in *Ms. Magazine*, recently [4]. Assuming no significant medical problem is evident in the pregnancy, as is still happily the usual case, the woman or couple still faces important choices. Under the time constraints of an advancing pregnancy, an obstetrical attendant must be chosen; though the woman may have an ongoing relationship with a gynecologist for routine care, pregnancy and the prospect of childbirth raise major questions not necessarily about competence, but about differences in style, philosophy and technique. It is possible in many parts of the country today to obtain prenatal care and natal care from a lay midwife, a certified nurse midwife, a general practitioner or family practitioner or a board certified obstetrician. Patients may deliver at home, in a hospital delivery room fully equipped for every medical emergency, or in an intermediate in-hospital or free-standing facility called an alternative birth center.

Facilities labeled birth centers range from those independent institutions which are equipped to deal only with low risk, low morbidity cases in which it is necessary to transfer complicated cases before or during labor to a hospital, to fully equipped hospital delivery rooms newly accoutered with curtains, pastel paint and champagne buckets. In response to strong consumer demands and economic pressures, most every hospital has seen fit to provide something called family-centered maternity care in some place called a 'birth center'. Determining the genuineness of a commitment beneath the label is a task far more complicated than finding the finest hospital in the city and is also reflected in the search for a physician or other birth attendant.

There are some genuine and central differences of opinion with regard to the practice of so-called normal obstetrics these days. Is childbirth a normal physiological event and the main thing to be avoided meddlesome midwifery or is childbirth an event fraught with hidden problems and the use of possibly invasive, or at least intrusive, diagnostic techniques more than justified by the morbidity and mortality avoided? The adherents of each school of thoughts use the welfare of the unborn baby to blackmail the expectant parents into submission. Although many practitioners profess moderation, each train of thought easily becomes a roller coaster from which it is very difficult to exit once the decision is made [13]. In addition, there are inherent contradictions between obstetric techniques proven or deemed valuable. For example, it has been amply demonstrated that physical activities such as walking during labor is associated with decreased pain and shortened time until delivery. However, until more advanced telemetry is developed, constant monitoring of uterine contactions and fetal heart tones demands considerable immobility. External monitors are not invasive but are uncomfortable and inaccurate. Fetal scalp monitors introduced through the vagina are less awkward and more precise. However, they require rupture of fetal membranes which commits the obstetrician to delivery within a matter of hours regardless of the progress of labor

Peripartum Care: Changes and Implications 97

in order to avoid uterine infection. Adherents of either system are quick to blame the parents who choose the other when anything goes awry. If friends, relatives and physician don't bring their responsibility to their attention the media or their lawyer will. How are parents to choose? The shelves of libraries and book stores are filled with childbirth preparation manuals of all sorts. Nearly everyone takes preparatory classes and those of the most popular teachers are filled 6 and 7 months before the due date of the couples enrolled. It is extremely difficult to predict which approach will work best for a given couple and how each practitioner and birth facility actually practices the philosophy it advertises [3]. The content of information in childbirth preparation classes ranges from an indoctrination to the hospital to counter-cultural admonitions on the avoidance of all medications and interventions. In defense of the latter position it must be said that no causal relationship between the improvement in obstetric outcome and the changes in obstetric techniques have been demonstrated. Some commonly used obstetrical techniques such as the lithotomy position for delivery are known to be detrimental to fetal circulation and the progress of labor; others, such as episiotomy, are practiced by virtue of tradition and belief, rather than any published studies to demonstrate their efficacy. Still others, such as ultrasound, appear promising, but await studies to document the safety over the long term of subjecting unborn babies to new modalities. In the middle of this situation stand the parents trying to master a new and bewildering situation and do the best for themselves and their baby.

They will attempt to sort out some of these choices in their childbirth classes. These classes taught to small groups of couples in the third trimester, usually by nurses or by specially trained childbirth educators, have some major common elements which constitute a small but significant social phenomenon of our time. Here for the first time, healthy young people gather voluntarily to learn about the physiology and psychology of a major life event. They practice techniques for lessening anxiety and pain by means of relaxation and distraction. They learn to support and communicate with each other and members of the health care team. They discover that many others in this situation have similar hopes and fears and feelings and possibly even helpful ways to deal with them. They learn about the advice given by other people's doctors and nurse-midwives. They learn to question authority in a constructive way and to practice for various potentially troublesome situations in labor and delivery. The involvement of fathers in this process is, to my knowledge, unprecedented in human history, but by and large their collaboration and presence is expected in upper middle class American society.

So modern day young couples may be more prepared for the reality of modern day hospital delivery than those of us who had children some years ago. The full enema and shave have largely disappeared. The father, or another close friend or relative in some cases, is in constant attendance, assisting with relaxation techniques and whispering encouragement. The laboring woman has an obligatory i.v. for purposes of hydration and the administration of any emergently required medication or blood. Labor is constantly monitored electronically. The intrauterine sounds may be broadcast softly into the room and the paper readout from the monitor may receive as much attention as the physical person of the mother [10]. Also in frequent attendance is a pumping devise for administering a constant infusion of epidural anesthesia during the latter stages of labor. In the 15 or 20 to even 40% of cases in which the readout from the fetal monitor is disturbing to the attendant, cesarean section will be performed. Parents who may be aware of cultural concern over the increase in the number of cesarean sections in recent years are in no position to quibble when the safety of their unborn child is said to be in jeopardy and the discomforts and anxieties of labor overwhelming.

Aside from the larger number of mothers recuperating from operative delivery, changes in postpartum care include shorter hospital stays for women after vaginal delivery (hours to a day or two in many cases), increased encouragement and practice of breast-feeding in the middle and upper middle classes, increased time spent by the normal baby at its mother's bedside rather than in the nursery and a bewildering array of interventions for the baby with complications, ranging from photo treatment for hyperbilirubinemia to highly developed neonatal intensive care and surgery [2]. In these units the baby may appear to its frightened parents as a tiny morsel of flesh connected to a myriad of clicking metal machines. In the case of a normal delivery, as mentioned above, the mother and infant will be sent home in short order with little professional supervision or chance to get acquainted beforehand [6]. At this point in 1984 more than half of the mothers of infants return to paid employment before their children are 6 months old. What psychological demands do these new developments place on people contemplating and undergoing the throes of parenthood? Although a wide range of circumstances has just been discussed, they share many psychological elements. First of all, new knowledge, new choices and new techniques, combined with consumer pressure for involvement (paradoxical though it may seem to have considered any woman 'uninvolved' in her own childbirth), combine to place great cognitive demands on individuals. In fact, informed decision-making is the law of the land. The information itself is complex, technical and sometimes beyond the bounds of ordinary contemplation (e. g. conception in a Petri dish). The same information may be conveyed with opposing emotional valences by equally persuasive social groups; for example, physician specialty groups and consumer self-help groups. Decisions must be made on the basis of the information despite the fact that the consequences of the alternatives are often not yet known in their entirety. In addition to the stress these cognitive demands place on the individual, they complicate important interpersonal relationships. Despite consumer complaints about arrogance and paternalism, authoritative, unambivalent and involved doctors have been sought by people in distress from time immemorial. Their emotional place cannot be filled by journal articles, legal decisions, laboratory technicians and machines and a succession of subspecialists.

Current mores also presuppose a high level of collaboration and cooperation between marital partners. We assume that the virtual exclusion of men from childbirth in nearly all known cultures was a mistaken preliminary to the enlightenment of today. Now both sexes are required to experience pregnancy and childbirth cognitively, psychologically and, insofar as possibly, physically, even when cesarean sections are performed. This calls for degrees of empathy, interpersonal communication skill and emotional resilience which may not be a part of everyone's basic equipment [14]. In the case of artificial insemination or surrogate motherhood, the situation also requires the biological absence of one of the parents and the biological presence of a third party in the family. Mishaps occasion the sharing of guilt not with a deity but with the collaborators in the decision. The resulting tension may well be a factor in the rising number of malpractice claims. Another possible factor and, in any event, a new psychological demand is the above-mentioned substitution of laboratory and technical care for the hands on care of the past. The invasion of the hitherto inviolate intrauterine space by the amniocentesis needle or the ultrasound scanner, the symbolic invasion of the marital bed by reproductive endocrinologists, the wires, strange noises and printouts of the fetal monitor, all are technical maneuvres which may be experienced by different individuals either as benign extensions of the helping professional or diabolical indicators of dire consequences.

These psychological demands and issues, as already hinted, have both advantages and disadvantages. The opportunity to know and to choose is an opportunity to master a social situation and a physiological event. As parenthood calls for great stores of empathy, emotional resilience, maturity, and tolerance for frustration, so it would seem advantageous to begin it with an experience of success. The sometimes difficult processes of information gathering and decision making, and the acceptance of ambiguity and conflict stand future parents in good stead, as does the childbirth preparation class experience of peer support and exchange, practice at dealing with authority figures and the acquisition of skills in the reduction of anxiety. The accessibility of detailed information about ones own anatomical and physiological functioning offers hope of cognitive grappling with disappointments and setbacks as in infertility cases. Advance knowledge of the sex of the baby long before it is born may enable its parents to prepare psychologically especially if the child will not be the sex they greatly desire. Advance knowledge that the baby does not suffer from a known genetic illness may make the second half of pregnancy much more pleasant for high-risk parents. Knowing that the fetus does suffer from a genetic abnormality enables the parents who wish to terminate the pregnancy to resolve the situation quickly. Even those who do not wish to terminate the pregnancy have sometimes commented that they appreciate the added months of warning time before they are confronted with the physical realities and needs of the neonate and the reactions of family and friends. Many couples state that their relationships were strengthened by the process of learning, deciding and experiencing either good or bad events together.

Health professionals and social scientists will note these positive sequelae with pleasure. However, we are more likely in our clinical work to be called upon to deal with the potential psychological pitfalls of recent developments as they interact with the psychodynamics of individual human beings. Let me cite some examples. The advent of amniocentesis as a routine measure in the care of large groups of patients is experienced by some of those patients at least as an impediment in the normal or usual development of attachment to the fetus by the pregnant women. Learning in the abstract that the child is not of the first choice gender without the external tangible reality of the child itself may lead to a crystallization of negative feelings which the usual sequence of events avoids. Some prospective parents, mothers especially, specifically request that the information be withheld for this reason. Case example: A young pregnant woman was already the mother of 2 sons. As her sister had already given birth to a son as well, the entire family was eager that she be delivered of a daughter on whom dolls and frilly dresses could be lavished. Nobody knew the sex of the baby before it was born. She delivered a third boy and wrote to a relative. 'When the doctor said "It is a boy" my heart fell, but then when I saw his little fat face and held him in my arms I fell in love with him.' An abstract boy was not so loveable as one who nestled at his mother's breast.

Styles and techniques of obstetrical care have changed so rapidly in recent decades that it is difficult for one generation to pass on any useful lore to the next. It is difficult for young women today, sometimes, to understand the passive stances taken by their mothers at the times of their own births. It is painful for grandfathers to contemplate their son's entry into the taboo inner sanctum – the delivery suite, and modern day fathers may have to cope with retrospective disappointment about the noninvolvement of their own fathers. These intergenerational gaps may be greater with couples who opt for so-called natural or noninterventive style of obstetrical care. High tech care is more consonant with the authoritarian hospital approach of 25–30 years ago.

The choices and conflicting information and wishes intrinsic in current developments make for a particular repeated style of miscommunication in interpersonal conflict. Here are some typical scenarios.

A patient comes in for her first prenatal visit and informs the obstetrician that she insists upon knowing risks, benefits and alternatives to any procedure contemplated. He agrees. Some months later at the appropriate time she goes into labor, but progress is not smooth. The doctor comes into the labor room to discuss the pros and cons of the enhancement of labor, the use of sedation and the possibility of cesarean section. The patient informs him, 'I'm exhausted, you're the doctor, you decide.' The doctor is uncertain as to what is the best course to follow with the patient at the moment and what the long-term ramifications of the alternative are. This scenario and the following one are so common as to warrant advance rehearsal by all pregnant families and their caretakers.

Case example: A couple prepare for the birth of their child by attending LaMaze classes. They practice relaxation exercises and breathing techniques together each evening after work. They agree that analgesic medication presents a danger to the child which is not worth the risk unless there are confounding complications and they look forward to meeting the challenge of labor together. At term there are two episodes of false labor resulting in hospital admission and discharge and much loss of sleep by both husband and wife. Finally, labor begins in earnest and good progress is made up to 6 or 7 cm. At this point the wife declares 'I've had enough of natural childbirth, please call the doctor and the nurse at once and insist that I be given some analgesia or anesthesia. I simply can't take it anymore.' The husband must make an on the spot decision whether to comply with this request or to view it as an expression of distress on the part of his wife which should be the signal for him to redouble his efforts to support her attempt to cope with her labor. In either case, it may seem afterwards that they were on the same wavelength so to speak, and the decision may feel mutual and supportive. However, in either case he runs a definite risk. He may intervene with the medical staff only to have his wife accuse him after birth of letting her down just when she needed him the most. She may feel robbed of her sense of mastery, tricked by the doctor and hospital, and guilty about the effects on her labor and her child. If only her husband had encouraged her as they planned and practiced, she could have made it on her own.

If, on the other hand, the husband opts for cognitive or emotional reasons to counter his wife's request for pharmacologic intervention with support and encouragement of her relaxation techniques, he runs a different risk. In this common scenario his wife greets him after delivery with accusations of callousness and abandonment. She informs him that when he has a baby he can tolerate all the involved sensations without pharmacologic aid, but that he has no right to withhold them from her in the face of her explicit request. How can he possibly know what agony she was suffering and how tired she was? Was he thinking only of the baby or of his triumphant reports to relatives, colleagues and the LaMaze class teacher? It will be a long time before there will be another baby in this family, etc. etc. In these cases, mother, father and medical staff may feel embittered and disaffected.

There are two last general issues that harken back to the anecdote at the beginning of the paper (the mother who complained about her contraceptive choices). The issues of guilt and disappointment run through the anecdotes just cited as well. With the scope of option, possibilities and treatable conditions broadening every day, there is a tendency to believe prematurely that if all involved parties make the right choices the desired and perfect result will always be attained. Expectations – for fertility, for pregnancy, for parenthood – are enormous. Adverse results lead to enormous disappointment and a search within and without for the responsible persons and behavior. When the blame is projected on to the reproductive partner, interpersonal strife results. Concerns about medical wrongdoing lead to malpractice suits. The almost inevitable review of ones own behavior and feelings with its equally inevitable discovery of lapses from the ideal, lead to shame and guilt. *Stewart* [14] describes 9 cases, 5 women and 4 men, who sought psychiatric treatment within 6 months of attempted natural childbirth. Complaints ranged from depression to anxiety, obsessive-compulsive behavior, phobic symptoms, and marital and sexual problems. While the bona fide effects of childbirth preparation and of other developments deserve or demand careful scientific scrutiny, we must not succumb to the temptation to blame all psychiatric symptomatology on them. Surely, childbirth itself and forms of intervention found at other times and in other places were associated with psychopathology as well. However, certain aspects of modern care do intensify the conflict of interest problem mentioned earlier. A pregnant or laboring woman, or even one who contemplates pregnancy, may feel she has to choose between being a martyr and being a child abuser. These are not pleasant or constructive alternatives. And they are especially difficult to bear in an era in which there are few peers or parents to share and understand ones experience and in which one expects perfection. It is important for experts in obstetrics and psychology to be aware of today's practices and their psychological implications. There are undoubtedly many more than can be mentioned, here, but they deserve the same careful attention as the blips on the fetal monitor or the daily rises and falls of the basal temperature.

One other point deserves mention. In addition to treating the symptomatic patients, both obstetrical and psychiatric professionals have been called upon to perform interventions and make decisions with profound ethical and psychological significance. What is our proper role in deciding who shall carry and who shall abort? Who shall be inseminated, who shall carry a child for hire, who is entitled to microsurgery? We must navigate between the roles of technician and judge. Our personal integrity, the role of our profession and the care of our patients is at stake.

Acknowledgement

I would like to thank *Colette McNicholas* for her help in the preparation of this manuscript.

References

1 Notman, M.T.; Nadelson, C.C. (ed.): The woman patient, medical and psychological interfaces, vol. 1: Sexual and reproductive aspects of women's health care (Plenum Press, New York 1978).
2 Leeuw, R. de: Neonatal intensive care – impact on families. J. psychosom. Obstet. Gynaec. *1:* 120 (1982).
3 Silvestre, D.; Fresco, N.: The insane notion of mastery over the body. J. psychosom. Obstet. Gynaec. *1:* 139 (1982).
4 Hubbard, R.: The fetus as patient, Ms. Magazine, p. 28, October 1982.
5 Annas, G.J.: Contracts to bear a child: compassion or commercialism? Hastings Center Rep., p. 23, April 1981.
6 Klaus, M.H.; Kennell, H.H.: Maternal-infant bonding (Mosby, St. Louis, 1976).
7 Wertz, R.W.; Wertz, D.C.: Lying-in. A history of childbirth in America (Schocken, New York 1979).
8 Colman, A.; Colman, L.: Pregnancy. The psychological experience (Bantam, New York 1971).
9 Berne-Framell, K.; Kjessler, B.; Josefson, G.: Anxiety concerning fetal malformations in women who accept or refuse alpha-fetoprotein screening in pregnancy. J. psychosom. Obstet. Gynaec. *2:* 94 (1983).
10 Jackson, J.E.; Vaughan, M.; Black, P.; D'Souze, S.W.: Psychological aspects of fetal monitoring: maternal reaction in the position of the monitor and staff behaviour. J. psychosom. Obstet. Gynaec. *2:* 97 (1983).
11 Fresco, N.; Silvestra, D.: The medical child: comments on prenatal diagnosis. J. psychosom. Obstet. Gynaec. 1: 3 (1982).
12 Kloosterman, G.J.: The universal aspects of childbirth: human birth as a socio-psychosomatic paradigm. J. psychosom. Obstet. Gynaec. *1:* 35 (1982).
13 Richards, M.P.M.: The trouble with 'choice' in childbirth. Birth *9:* 253 (1982).
14 Stewart, D.E.: Psychiatric symptoms following attempted natural childbirth. Can. med. Ass. J. *127:* 713 (1982).
15 AAP and ACOG Statement on Alpha Fetoprotein Testing. New Release, The American College of Obstetricians and Gynecologists (Washington, DC, 1983).
16 Hobbins, J.C.: Determination of fetal sex in early pregnancy. New Engl. J. Med. *309:* 979 (1983).

N.L. Stotland, MD, Pritzker School of Medicine, University of Chicago,
Psychiatric Liaison to Obstetrics and Gynecology, Michael Reese Hospital,
Chicago, IL 60616 (USA)

A View of Artificial Insemination

Elisabeth C. Small, R. Nuran Turksoy

Departments of Psychiatry and Obstetrics and Gynecology, University of Nevada, School of Medicine, Reno, Nev.; Department of Obstetrics and Gynecology, Tufts University School of Medicine, and Department of Obstetrics and Gynecology, Tufts New England Medical Center Hospital, Boston, Mass., USA

Although infertility is not usually considered to be a disease state, it can be the source of a great deal of psychic pain and disappointment to couples with hopes of building a family. The estimation of infertile marriages in the United States is 1 in 10, and of these 40–50% are entirely or partially due to male factors [1]. For some infertile couples, artificial insemination, when performed with skill and utmost care in selection, may offer a possible solution to their unhappiness.

Artificial insemination, or artificial impregnation, is the process by which a female is brought to conception without intravaginal coition. This is effected by the deposition of semen into the vaginal canal, the cervix, or the uterus. In cases where the semen is taken from the husband, the process is called artificial insemination, homologous (AIH). When the semen is procured from a male other than the husband, the terms artificial insemination by donor (AID) or heterologous insemination are used. Other terms for donor insemination are therapeutic insemination or semiadoption. In some instances where the husband's semen is mixed with donor semen, the process is termed biseminal artificial insemination (BAI).

The most recent development in fertilization technique has been that of in vitro fertilization for women in whom both fallopian tubes have been surgically removed or destroyed by infection. In this situation the husband's sperm is used to fertilize the ovum which is recovered from the woman's ovary during the ovulatory phase of her cycle. Then the fertilized ovum, at the appropriate stage of development, can be implanted into the woman's uterus, during the same ovulatory cycle. Successful results have already been reported.

In the veterinary literature, artificial insemination dates back to the 14th century when mention is made of Arabs who impregnated mares of their enemies with semen of inferior stallions. The first published paper on the subject was written by the Abbé *Lazarro Spallanzani* in 1784, describing fertilization of a dog and other animals [2]. Large scale use of artificial insemination was stimulated by *Iwanow,* the Russian physiologist whose distinguished monograph described the process in 1907 [3].

The advantages of the uses of artificial insemination in animal husbandry are now unquestioned. Since 1930, the rapid increase of its use in livestock breeding is particularly noted in the dairy industry, where it is now applied to nearly 99% of cows in the more economically advanced countries. Other mammals inseminated by this means include ewes, sows, mares, goats, and in lesser numbers, the domestic dog and cat [4].

Earliest documentation of artificial insemination of a human occurred in 1793 in the case of a linen draper in London who suffered from hypospadias and required that his wife be inseminated with his collected semen by *John Hunter.* This developed into a normal pregnancy and was reported in 1799 by *Home* [5]. In 1866, *J.M. Sims* reported artificial insemination done on 6 wives, each using the husband's semen. 1 patient became pregnant, but later aborted the first successful artificial insemination performed in the United States. Though *Sims* was initially enthusiastic about the procedure, he later condemned both the procedure and his own part in it on the grounds that it was an immoral medical practice. In the early 20th century, German workers continued to attempt husband inseminations with some reported successes [6,7].

In the United States the first case of human donor insemination performed in 1884 was reported by *A.D. Hard* in 1909 in a paper entitled 'Artificial Impregnation'. This case caused a great deal of controversy in the medical community, the argument being that the artificial insemination was not itself unknown, but obtaining semen and then inseminating it was considered 'ridiculously criminal' and may be considered disrespectful to the laws of Nature and of God [8]. Arguments such as these still persist, but through the efforts of study by the early American workers, *R.L. Dickinson* and *W. Carey,* donor insemination has become a rational method for treating sterility in certain selected cases.

Since the mid-1960s, demand for the AID procedure has been greatly increased because of the difficulty in the treatment of male infertility and the marked decrease in the number of babies available for adoption. It is impossible to detemine how many babies are born annually as a result of donor insemination, since records of AID are usually held in secrecy. *Guttmacher* [9] estimated in 1961 that approximately 5000–7000 artificially inseminated babies are born per year in the United States. This is considered by many current workers to be a very conservative estimate and a figure between 10 000 and 250 000 has also been given.

Religious Aspects

There is a wide range of religious opinion regarding artificial insemination. All authorities in the Roman Catholic church, from Pope Leo XIII, condemn artificial insemination on the basis that the exclusive rights to procreation reside only in the marriage; that artificial insemination reduces man to the level of animals and that the process is a grave threat to society. In 1949, Pope Pius XII had further statement of artificial insemination by donor: 'Who ever gives life to little human beings, receives from nature herself, in virtue of that very relationship, the responsibility of its conservation and education. But between the lawful husband and the child who is the fruit of an active element derived from a third party (even should the husband consent) there is no link of origin, no moral and juridical bond of conjugal procreation...'.

In 1948, a 13-member commission appointed by the Archbishop of Canterbury to study artifical insemination was inconclusive in their report on AIH but rendered a decision of firmly opposing donor insemination, laying emphasis on the question of adultery, on the secrecy surrounding the process and the necessity for the falsification of records. The one dissenting vote by Dean *Matthews* of St. Paul expressed his concern that a judgment on such an imperfectly understood matter was premature [10]. Other Protestant denominations have made no official stand and are noncommittal, with no objection where biological and moral precautions are considered.

Most rabbinic opinion regarding artificial insemination by donor other than husband considers the process to be an abomination and it is strictly prohibited on the grounds of the possibility of incest, lack of genealogy, and the problems of inheritance. Some authorities regard insemination as adultery, but much rabbinic opinion states that without a sexual act involved, the woman is not guilty of adultery and can cohabit with the husband. A child conceived by donor is considered legitimate. A husband whose wife bears a donor-inseminated child with or without his permission may sue for divorce but is not required to do so. The reform Jewish rabbinic authorities tend to be more accepting in insemination than those of the orthodox.

Rabbinic opinions usually sanction use of the husband's sperm after a 5- to 10-year waiting period where pregnancy cannot be achieved in any other way. Here, question is raised as to the method of sperm collection. Self-stimulation (masturbation) is not condoned, but natural intercourse with condom or coitus interruptus is less objectionable. In general, opinion is that an act performed for the sole purpose of making possible a birth can never be regarded as an offense whether or not the precept of procreation is thereby technically carried out [11].

Legal Aspects

There are no uniform laws passed by the separate states in the United States, nor are there any national laws regarding artificial insemination. Furthermore, there are no laws which make artificial insemination illegal whether by husband or by donor. Essentially, AIH raises no legal problems since it is performed with consent of husband and wife and involves no extramarital factors. On the other hand, donor insemination introduces an individual who must remain anonymous to husband and wife and as a result AID involves 5 or possibly 6 individuals, each with rights and responsibilities. These include husband, wife, doctor, donor, child, and occasionally the donor's wife. The major issues which are raised include that of adultery and the legal status and rights of the child [12].

In the case of adultery, criminal adultery cannot occur in the absence of sexual intercourse, since criminal statutes are to be strictly construed. Thus, when the statute involved does not specifically include AID, it seems unlikely that an action of criminal adultery would arise. However, in civil cases of divorce, the courts are divided as to whether AID constitutes adultery. Under English law, 2 people must be together, physically engaged in the sexual act at the same time, and there must be sexual intercourse to constitute adultery. When such does not exist, there is no adultery. This is considered the best course of reasoning for American courts to follow.

The most important and far-reaching issue concerns the child. In the United States, several states have established the legitimacy of the child conceived by donor insemination (California, Connecticut, Georgia, Kansas, New York, North Carolina, Oklahoma, and Texas). Most decisions also entitle the child to support from the mother's husband, at least when he has consented to the AID process, unless adultery is proven in court. The husband, in turn, is entitled to visitation rights. A statute enacted in New York, effective May 7, 1974, establishes that a child born through artificial insemination is deemed to be legitimate and the natural child of the husband and wife for all purposes if: (1) the child is born to a married woman; (2) the artificial insemination is performed by persons duly authorized to practice medicine, and (3) the written consent of both the woman and her husband is obtained. The written consent is to be executed and acknowledged by husband and wife. The physician performing the insemination must certify that he or she rendered the service. In addition, court decisions now tend to defend the inheritance rights of children issuing from consensual AID without the added legal procedure of adoption. It is worthwhile for the physician to know the legal status of AID in his or her state.

Contingent to the legitimacy issue is the problem of the birth certificate. It is considered to be perjury if a physician knowingly inserts the husband's name on the birth certificate of a child conceived by AID. To obviate this difficulty, many physician-inseminators do not give obstetrical service to their recipients, but refer the patient to an obstetrician who, unaware of the insemination, can sign the birth certificate as he would with any routine delivery, with the husband identified as father of the child.

There are other questions about the liability of the physician as well as the donor. Can the physician be held liable for support if the husband has not given consent? Such may be an excessive liability, and perhaps a monetary penalty would be preferable if a legislature wished to discourage nonconsensual AID. Certainly AID without consent from the recipient would be unprivileged touching and would constitute battery. To hold a donor liable for support would presuppose exposing his identity and would be a problem if records were not properly kept. Donor consent and consent from the donor's wife is suggested to avoid potential problems, especially that of finding a donor guilty of adultery where his wife's consent was not obtained [13].

Artificial insemination of single women and lesbian women is being performed in some clinics. Because of the increasing rate of divorce, many children are raised by mothers who have been awarded custody. Widows also raise children alone. The argument in favor of inseminating the unmarried women lies in the fact that here has been no clear-cut evidence that children who are raised by a single parent suffer more emotional or physical damage than those children who are not. The matter is under much controversy and carried with it further legal and ethical questions. In England, where lesbian women have been inseminated, the British Medical Association has left it for the physician to consider each case individually, taking into consideration the welfare of the patient and also weighing the effects on the child. Most physicians will not inseminate a woman when they know that the baby will have no father. It is felt that the child in this situation would have no chance to experience an intact family structur, and would be thus entering an unstable environment.

The Process of Artificial Insemination

Artificial insemination by husband is considered for couples who have mechanical difficulties in achieving coitus, or in couples where the husband has subnormal reproductive ability. Insemination by donor is considered in cases of infertility in the male, in situations where the husband carries a genetic factor which makes for abnormal offspring, or where there is an Rh-negative wife who has been sensitized by an Rh-positive husband and who has borne a succession of hydropic infants.

The general process of evaluation of an infertile couple for artificial insemination begins with a thorough evaluation of the couple consisting of physical examination, diagnostic tests, and psychological evaluation.

The social and psychological aspect of the insemination process canot be overemphasized. *Guttmacher* [9] offers a set of ground rules which include the advice that the physician know the couple, ascertain their intellectual capacity and emotional stability, and if possible, the likelihood of a permanent marriage. He feels that only a small percentage of couples applying qualify for so radical a procedure. A psychiatrist can be used for this aspect of the evaluation.

Collection and Storage of Sperm

Semen from the male, be he the husband or the donor, is collected after self-stimulation. The male produces the ejaculate into a small wide-mouthed sterile plastic or glass jar. The semen, ejaculated in liquid form, becomes a gel or coagulum immediately after ejaculation. It liquefies again within 5–20 min. Subsequently it can be drawn up into a sterile syringe and be ready for use. For husbands who cannot self-stimulate to ejaculation, the use of condom collection or coitus interruptus can be used as an alternative. However, this type of collection does not provide good specimens for insemination.

Timing of semen collection and the optimum time for insemination do not usually coincide. Furthermore, there are few centers performing artificial insemination and patients often travel considerable distances. The availability of stored semen offers an advantage when dealing with a problem as variable as female ovulation [12].

Frozen semen has been used in animal husbandry for many years, but in human use, preservation and frozen storage of semen has only been gradually increased in the past 20 years. If frozen semen can be preserved without change in fertility and damage in embryo development, it offers much more flexibility to the process of artificial insemination. There has been particular consideration in the possibility of semen storage in men contemplating vasectomy or chemotherapy and radiation therapy for malignant diseases. This issue of fertility insurance must be handled with caution. It is impossible to anticipate and guarantee every fertile male that his semen may remain fertile after years of storage. In some cases, by human error, semen may be damaged or lost. The problem of use of semen stored after a man has died either by disease or natural causes also raises ethical and legal questions and the possibility of the upset of the balance of the sexes.

Insemination Techniques

There are four basic types of insemination procedures: intravaginal, cervicovaginal, intrauterine, and the use of a cervical cap. In practice, the cervicovaginal and the intrauterine methods are the most commonly used.

AIH

The effectiveness of AIH in unselected cases is open to question. In selected cases, if the treatment is carried out skillfully, the method holds a good chance of success. AIH should not be utilized as a last resort of therapy in cases of infertility where the etiology is obscure. Indications of its use must be clear. Artificial insemination using the husband's semen is of significant value only in those instances where seminal delivery by the husband during sexual intercourse is not possible.

The success rate of AIH can be divided into three groups. Those groups which have the highest success fall into the following situations: (1) instances of penile deformities such as hypospadias which can cause deposition of sperm outside the vagina, (2) abnormalities of coitus resulting from marked obesity, dyspareunia, vaginitis, vaginal strictures, or narrowing of the vaginal fornices and hood configurations around the cervix as a result of exposure to diethylstilbestrol (DES) during intrauterine life; (3) premature ejaculation or in instances of retrograde ejaculation, which is not an uncommon sequel after prostate surgery; (4) neurologic or psychological impotence refractory to treatment in cases where the husband cannot ejaculate in the vagina, but can give a specimen by self-stimulation; (5) use of frozen stored semen of good quality, which had been obtained from the husband prior to vasectomy, chemotherapy, or radiotherapy for malignancy.

Less successful results occur if the husband's semen production is abnormal as in the following conditions.

(1) The volume of semen may be too small or too large. If the semen analysis reveals a small volume of semen (less than 2 cm^3) but otherwise has normal characteristics, and the postcoital test shows no sperm in the cervical mucus un the presence of adequate intromission, AIH increases the chances of conception. Proper placement of semen at the cervical opening (os) prevents loss of semen into the vagina and ensures that the semen is in contact with the cervical mucus.

If the volume of semen is too large, the ejaculate can be separated into two parts (split ejaculate) during semen collection. In this technique, the first few drops of ejaculate are collected in one jar and the rest in a second jar. The first portion of the ejaculate contains the sperm-rich fractions and prostatic fluid. The remainder of the ejaculate which originates in the seminal vesicles can be harmful to the sperm in some males. The first fraction, with its greater concentration of sperm of better motility and less viscosity, is then used.

In cases where the couple may object to the collection of sperm by self-stimulation, the couple may use an alternative technique by themselves. During intercourse, the husband can withdraw as soon as he feels that ejaculation has begun. This in vivo technique has been successfully practiced by some couples and pregnancies from this method have been reported [14].

(2) The quality or quantity of the sperm may be abnormal: oligospermia (sperm count of less than 30 million/cm^3) and hypomotility (where activity of the sperm is less than 40%). The results of AIH with oligospermia and even in cases of borderline hypomotility have been generally poor. Since a low sperm count is frequently associated with other morphologic and biochemical abnormalities of the ejaculate, the fractional separation of

ejaculate will not be helpful in improving the biological quality of the semen.

AIH has the least success, but is of some value, in infertility caused by immunologic factors, resulting in the formation of antibodies.

(3) Antibodies against the sperm may prevent fertilization. These antibodies may be present in the wife's serum and secreted in the cervical mucus, or may be present in the husband's serum. Presence of antisperm antibodies can be detected by means of various immunologic tests in laboratories of specialized infertility clinics. Circulating antibodies in women usually disappear after 3–6 months of condom therapy, where use of a condom prevents cervical contact with the seminal contents and thus prevents antibody production. Following therapy, fertilization may be successful. In rare instances, conception may occur with the presence of antibodies.

(4) Autoantibodies prevent fertilization. In some instances, antibody production in the male may occur against his own sperm. This can be treated successfully by immunosuppressive therapy using steroids. Disappearance of these autoantibodies and subsequent pregnancies have been observed in some couples [15,16].

The overall success rate in AIH procedures per se does not exceed 30–35%.

Psychological Aspects of AIH

In most cases, the phenomenon of conception by AIH, if it occurs, is not far from that of normal coital insemination where no third party, other than the physician, is involved. AIH is less psychologically traumatic to the couple than is AID. Since there is hope and possibility that his fertility is still intact, the husband feels less anxious about his self-esteem and masculinity when going through this procedure which is designed to enhance his fertility.

There is no question that a thorough sexual history is an integral part of the workup to discover problems which may affect the need for insemination. Couples who are suffering from psychogenic impotence, premature ejaculation, vaginismus, or excessive obesity require further psychiatric evaluation and may require treatment before insemination. The sexual dysfunction can be a defense against the fear of reproduction and the responsibility of offspring. For example, a woman with vaginismus may be unconsciously protecting herself from impregnation and a pregnancy may be the farthest thing from her true wish. Insemination in this case is inviting disaster for the child as well as the parents. Some men who are impotent with their wives may have conflicts in the relationship or may have homosexual inclinations. These factors need to be well understood prior to insemination. Successful treatment of the psychological impediments to coitus may eliminate the necessity for artificial insemination.

On the other hand, there are also reports that some couples who have had success with AIH have been able to have coitus subsequently [17]. The cause of their infertility is clearly due to sexual dysfunction and not subfertility. Although there is usually a small chance of success in the use of AIH in chronically infertile couples, many oligospermic couples choose to attempt a series of treatments before accepting AID, and the experience of AIH is an effective introduction to the concept of donor insemination.

AID

Artificial insemination by donor is considered in cases of male steriity such as azoospermia (no sperm) or oligospermia (few sperm), proven by careful evaluation, and in situations where germ plasm carries catastrophic effect on the offspring such as the situation in Rh incompatibility between the couple or in cases where genetic factors lead to serious defects such as Tay-Sachs disease and Huntington's chorea.

Document of Agreement

The process in AID, after a medical and psychological evaluation, begins with an open discussion and full explanation of the medical, legal, ethical, and psychological aspects of the process. Often, a contractual agreement to the procedure is required, denoting the willingness of both parties to the insemination, as well as the acceptance of a child born by this method as a legitimate heir for whom both father and mother are responsible for support and care. The parents cannot disclaim the child as their own. The selection of the donor is left to the discretion of the physician, noting that there will be mutual anonymity between the donor and the couple. In essence, the couple makes a request for insemination, having discussed and understood what is involved and absolving the physician from any and every responsibility or complication from such a procedure [18]. While such a document may prevent law suits, the agreement by no means makes the procedure legal in the eyes of the law.

The practical aspects should be explained in detail. In our clinic the use of an anatomical model and the insemination tools are shown to the couple in the discussion. The possibility of success is also explained, as many couples are under the impression that the process is some sort of magic which will be unquestionably successful.

Selection of the Donor

Most clinics select only medical students, dental students, or young physicians as donors. An interview with the donor requires that he be informed of his role as donor, of the rule of anonymity, and the professional aspect of donorship by the fact that he is paid, usually in cash. The donor is not entitled to any further information about the results of the use of his sperm. A careful medical and eugenic family history follows. Use of medical students is considered to facilitate a more thorough history taking as the donors have a better understanding of the implications of the medical and genetic factors.

The requirements of the donor are that:

(1) He is healthy and intelligent. (Jewish donors are screened for Tay-Sachs disease.)

(2) He has proven fertility with semen of high quality: high concentration of sperm (greater than 80 million/cm^3; excellent motility (greater than 80%); normal morphology (60%), and adequate semen (2.5–5.0 cm^3 volume).

(3) He must be free of venereal disease and drug abuse.

(4) He must have matching physical caracteristics with the husband such as height, weight, build, color of hair and eyes, and complexion. Usually no attempts are made to duplicate race or religious backgrounds, but social and intellectual factors are taken into consideration.

(5) He must have a matching blood Rh grouping with the recipient.

Because of donor anonymity, fears of consanguinity have often been raised. The rare possibility that donor inseminated children may unwittingly marry other children of the same donor is remote, but has been reported. To avoid this possibility, it is advised that the number of babies fathered by a single donor remain small.

Procedure of Donor Insemination

In our clinic, the woman is instructed to keep a basal body temperature chart for a least 2 months before the insemination cycle. Patency of tubes is also documented by injection of dye into the uterus under fluoroscopic X-ray procedure (hysterosalpingogram) during this observation period. The best time for the insemination procedure is just prior to the time of ovulation (before the basal temperature rises). The cervical mucus secretion is a good indicator of estrogen secretion and is considered the best clinical index for optimal timing of insemination. The quantity of cervical mucus secretion correlates best with the preovulatory estrogen surge. If the cervical mucus secretion is not adequate on the planned insemination day, insemination ist postponed until the following day. An average of 2 inseminations per cycle is performed.

To facilitate the procedure and to predict the ovulation time more accurately, most physicians use Clomid (an ovulation-inducing drug) in standard doses. Usually, 50 mg of Clomid (1 tablet) is given for 5 days, starting on the 5th day of the menstrual cycle. Ovulation usually occurs 6–8 days after taking the last Clomid pill. Insemination is performed on the 5th and 6th days after the last Clomid administration (immediately prior to predicted ovulation).

The procedure of AID is relatively simple. The most suitable donor for each couple is selected. The identities of the couple and the donor are kept in great secrecy. In the clinic laboratory prior to the insemination, the donor produces a sample of semen which is collected and examined. The insemination takes place in another area, within 0.5 h of collection and examination, usually in the doctor's examining room. The husband is expected to accompany his wife during the procedure and to stay with her in the room after the insemination takes place.

The patient lies on an examination table with her pelvis slightly elevated. A sterile speculum is inserted into the vagina and the cervix is exposed. The semen sample, in small amounts, is injected gently into the cervical os through a plastic tube. The rest of the semen is injected onto the lower blade of the speculum so that the cervical os is covered with semen. The patient remains in this position for 30–40 min. It has been shown that the spermatozoa gain access to the fallopian tube within 15 min. In 45 min. the maximum number of spermatozoa will have reached the fallopian tube.

Results of AID

The overall success rate with AID in properly selected couples is about 70%. Of those women who achieve pregnancy, 95% conceive during the first 6 months of AID treatment. The abortion rate in these cases is the same as the general population. There is no increase in the congenital defects of babies born of these pregnancies. There is no proven scientific method for preselection of the sex of the baby.

Frozen sperm is utilized in some infertility clinics where fresh semen cannot be obtained. The commercially available frozen bank semen can be shipped to the physician's office on request. The physical characteristics of the donor and the quality of the semen are recorded on an accompanying data sheet.

In order to detect the presence of infection, cultures of the semen hab been otained prior to freezing. The motility of sperm can be impaired during the thawing of semen prior to insemination. The pregnancy ratio is somewhat lower than that of fresh semen. There is an hypothesis that the incidence of congenital anomalies in the offspring is lower than that found in the general population since the abnormal spermatozoa are eliminated due to their inability to withstand freezing [19].

Psychological Aspects of AID

Although it is generally accepted that in infertile couples the male is the reason in one third of the cases, there is a universal belief that barrenness is purely a women's perogative. When men are asked to provide a specimen of semen as a preliminary to the usual fertility study, a man's response is usually one of disbelief. This attitude may be grounded in biblical tradition where there are many references to barren women, and none to barren men. Added to this is the story of Sarah, childless, who urged Abraham to impregnate the servant Hagar (Genesis 16), thus recording the outcome of the first biological investigation of male fertility. These factors could explain the reason for the male's unquestionable belief in his own fertility [20].

The fact of irreversible male infertility destroys this belief, and understandably, the discovery of his own infertility shakes a man's self-esteem, self-worth, and sense of masculinity. Correction of one or more female factors is easier for a couple to accept than is the only alternative for an infertile male artificial insemination by sperm of another male. This fact differentiates the type of emotional response of AID from that of AIH.

Though the literature is sparse regarding the emotional aspects of AID, some studies are available which attempt to investigate the motivation and the emotional impact on individuals who have undergone donor insemination. *Farris' and Garrison's* [21] study of well-educated middle-class couples revealed that the most common conscious motivations of couples who choose AID over adoption include the desire to experience pregnancy. Women wanted to bear a child of their own and would have felt cheated without the experience; men desired the biological experience for the gratification of the wife. Couples were unwilling to choose adoption because they were dissatisfied with the adoption procedure, because they wished to avoid the stigma of adoption on the child, and because they felt that for the grandparents a child by insemination would be more acceptable than an adopted child.

The benefits derived from maternity included the sense that 50% known heredity was better than none, that genetic factors were under better control, and that the child would be more nearly theirs. Couples felt that they would have a closer emotional relationship to the infant in having shared the pregnancy experience form the beginning. Some couples, in the secrecy of the process, could conceal the infertility of the father from the public. More importantly, the husbands felt it would conceal a deficiency in themselves by concealing their sterility. Wives were primarily concerned with protecting their husbands and thereby indirectly concealing their own sense of shame.

For those couples whose religious backgrounds are associated with a denunciation of artificial insemination as immoral or adulterous, or a condemnation of masturbation, unconscious guilt can produce conflict.

Clinical observations reveal that the female usually has no great discomfort in donor insemination. The woman is seldom bothered by a sense of invasion of her body, and actually may feel satisfaction in the procedure. If she is successfully impregnated, she may feel a sense of superiority as well as a sense of fulfillment. If a woman is at all hesistant to undergo the treatment, it may be that she is concerned about her husband's sense of vulnerability and is uncertain that he can make a successful adjustment to having a child in this fashion [22]. Some women, in refusing adoption, may be unwilling to endure with their husbands the mutual frustration of not being able to create a child. Being unable to mourn the shared loss of reproductivity, the wife may demand the gratification of her need to bear a child no matter what the damaging effects may be on the relationship with the man she expects to help raise the child. The motivations of women for pregnancy are well discussed by *Nadelson* [23].

The male, on the other hand, knows of his responsibility in the problem and feels not only his own disappointment, but also feels the sadness of his wife's frustrations. Consequently, feelings of inadequacy, inferiority, and guilt can result. Some husbands who react to the idea of AID as unacceptable may see the procedure as somewhat better than adultery. If their wives become pregnant, feelings of biological deficiency may surface and they may develop jealousy of the anonymous donor or develop resentment toward the child. However, there are those who are not distressed by the addition of a third part, and are able to share with their wives in the emotional gratifications of the pregnancy and welcome the child as their own.

In the usual situation, a man must overcome his initial resistance to AID, but will agree to it for the sake of making his wife happy, to obtain a child which he desires, to relieve feelings of guilt, and to conceal his infertility. In a successful adjustment, he becomes as eager as his wife to have the insemination. Though his motives are usually sincere, even a careful psychological evaluation cannot predict a change to negative feelings of resentment, anger, and repudiation at some future crisis.

There are case reports of maladaptive aspects of donor insemination [24,25] and some isolated cases of psychosis following AID. However, there are as yet no large scale reported systematic psychological studies of AID couples and their offspring. What data is available is mostly retrospective and utilizes mainly the anonymous questionnaire, or occasional physician contact with the patient. The general observations from such studies are: (1) that marriages usually do not deteriorate [18,26,27]; (2) the couples are happy, grateful, and feel close to the children whom they consider their own [26,28,29], and (3) when queried whether they would consider having another child by the same method, the response is predominately in the affirmative and many couples to return for further inseminations [21,26,29–31].

Effects on Children of AID

The confines of secrecy and anonymity to protect the children of AID have also excluded them from observation. There is only one reported study on children of AID. This is a report from Japan which revealed that measurements of mental development (intelligence quotient and developmental quotient) and physical development (height and weight) were greater than that of a control group of naturally inseminated children. Of the 54 children in the study, 9 were the results of insemination by frozen semen [32].

The technique of artificial insemination is relatively simple, but because of its unnatural character, complex issues of moral, legal, social, and psychological consequences are raised. It is the responsibility of the physician and the infertile couple to be cognizant of these issues and to utilize utmost care in arriving at the decision to use the procedure for the purpose of bringing health and happiness to the couple themselves, to the resultant child and to society as a whole.

References

1 Speroff, L.; Glass, R. H.; Kass, N. G.: Clinical gynecologic endocrinology and infertility; 2nd ed., p. 363. (Williams & Wilkins, Baltimore, 1978).
2 Spallanzani, L.: Dissertations relative to the natural history of animals and vegetables; translated from the Italian of the Abbé Spallanzani (Murray, London, 1784).
3 Iwanow, E.J.: De la fécundation artificielle chez les mammifères. Archs Sci. biol., St. Petersburg, Russia *12:* 377 (1907).
4 Jones, R. C.: Uses of artificial insemination. Nature, Lond. *229:* 534–537 (1971).
5 Home, E.: An account of the dissection of a hermaphrodite dog, etc. Phil. Trans. R. Soc. Lond. *89:* 157 (1799).
6 Frankel, L.: Über künstliche Befruchtung beim Menschen und ihre gerichtsärztliche Beurteilung. Ärztl. SachverstZtg. *15:* 169 (1909).
7 Döderlein, A.: Über künstliche Befruchtung. Münch. med. Wschr. *59:* 1081 (1912).
8 Gregoire, A.T.; Mayer, R. C.: The impregnators. Fert. Steril. *16:* 130–134 (1965).
9 Guttmacher, A.F.: The role of artificial insemination in the treatment of sterility. Obstetl. gynec. Surv. *15:* 767–785 (1960).
10 Levisohn, A.A.: Dilemma in parenthood. J. forens. Med. *4:* 147 (1957).
11 Rosner, F.: Sperm procurement and analysis in Jewish law. Am. J. Obstet. Gynec. *130:* 627–629 (1978).
12 Beck, W.W.: A critical look at the legal, ethical and technical aspects of artificial insemination. Fert. Steril. *27:* 1–8 (1976).
13 Pecklins, D.M.: Artificial insemination and the law. J. legal Med. July/August *1976:* 17–22.
14 Amelar, R.D.; Hotchkiss, R.S.: The split ejaculate: its use in the management of male infertility. Fert. Steril. *16:* 46–60 (1965).
15 Shulman, S.: Treatment of immune male infertility with methylprednisone. Lancet *ii:* 1243 (1976).
16 Dondero, F.; Isidoro, A.; Lenzi, A.; et al: Treatment and follow-up of patients with infertility due to spermagglutins. Fert. Steril. *31:* 48–51 (1979).
17 Russel, J.K.: Artificial insemination (husband) in the management of childlessness. Lancet *ii:* 1223 (1960).
18 Behrman, S.J.: Techniques of artificial insemination; in Behrman, Kistner, Progress in infertility, pp. 717–730. (Little, Brown, Boston 1968).
19 Steinberger, E.; Smith, K.D.: Artificial insemination with fresh or frozen semen, a comparativ study. J. Am. med. Ass. *223:* 778–783 (1973).
20 An obstetrician: Barrenness – the woman's perogative? S. Afr. med. J. *50:* 871–872 (1976).
21 Farris, E.J.; Garrison, M.J.: Emotional impact of successful donor insemination. Obstet. Gynec., N.Y. *3:* 19–20 (1954).
22 Lamson, H.D.; Pinard, W.J.; Meaker, S.R.: Sociologic and psychological aspects of artificial insemination with donor semen. J. Am. med. Ass. *145:* 1062–1064 (1951).
23 Nadelson, C.C.: 'Normal' and 'Special' aspects of pregnancy: a psychological approach; in Notman, Nadelson, The woman patient, vol. 1: Sexual and reproductive aspects of women's health care, pp. 73–86. (Plenum Press, New York, 1979).

24 Gerstel, G.: A psychoanalytic view of artificial donor insemination. Am. J. Psychother. *17:* 64–77 (1963).
25 Watters, W.W.; Sousa-Poza, J.: Psychiatric aspects of artificial insemination (donor). Can. med. Ass. J. *95:* 106–113 (1966).
26 Levie, L.H.: An inquiry into the psychological effects on parents of artificial insemination with donor semen. Eugen. Rev. *59:* 97–105 (1967).
27 Langer, G.; Lemberg, E.; Sharf, M.: Artificial insemination: a study of 156 succesful cases. Int. J. Fert. *14:* 232–240 (1969).
28 Løvset, J.: Artificial insemination: the attitude of patients in Norway. Fert. Steril. *2:* 415–429 (1951).
29 Simmons, F.A.: Role of the husband in therapeutic donor insemination. Fert. Steril *8:* 547–550 (1957).
30 Warner, M.P.: Artificial insemination: review after 32 years' experience. N. Y. St. J. Med. *74:* 2358–2361 (1974).
31 David, A.; Avidan, D.: Artificial insemination donor: clinical and psychological aspects. Fert. Steril. *27:* 528–532 (1976).
32 Iizuka, R.; Sawada, Y.; Nishina, N.; Ohi, M.: The physical and mental development of children born following artificial insemination. Int. J. Fert. *13:* 24–32 (1968).

Addendum:
In vitro Fertilization, Embryo Transfer and Surrogate Parenting

A discussion of artificial insemination cannot exclude some commentary on the newest attempts of treating infertility by in vitro fertilization, embryo transfer or the use of surrogates. Although little data are yet available regarding the social, emotional and legal consequences of these modalities, there are considerations to be included in the use of any of these treatments.

The in vitro fertilization technique was developed by *Patrick Steptoe* and *Robert Edwards* of Great Britain, resulting in the first successful birth by this method in 1978. The method involves the laparoscopic removal of an ovum immediately before ovulation, its incubation in a Petri dish with washed and centrifugated ejaculate from a male. Induction of ovulation by Clomid may or may not be utilized. Incubation of the embryo is continued to the blastocyst stage and subsequently is transported into the uterus by pipette. If the embryo is successfully implanted, then the production of choriogonadotropins occurs, menstruation ceases and gestation continues. The possibility of freezing spare embryos for the donation to infertile women has also received attention, but is not yet a frequent practice [1]

Use of surrogate mothers allows for the artificial insemination of the surrogate by the semen of the husband of an infertile pair. She can carry the pregnancy to term and give the child up to the couple after delivery. In situations of embryo transfer, a surrogate may also receive and gestate a fertilized in vitro ovum, or give up an in vivo fertilized ovum to a woman desiring a pregnancy, who has either tubal or hereditary disorder problems. Male donors cannot only provide semen for artificial insemination as previously described, but also can donate semen for in vitro insemination in situations of male factor infertility. In cases where either husband or wife may have hereditary disorders which the couple do not wish to propagate, then selection of a third party, either male or female, to provide the gamete is no longer a difficult issue. The new technology has arrived at allowing women to carry a biologically unrelated child or a frozen embryo to term.

Results of the advances in reproductive techniques give rise to variations of parenthood depending on the number and identities of donors, recipients and the parenting couple. However, the legal problem of rights and responsibility have not kept pace in development. Not only is the legitimacy of the child (even with the husband's consent) still an open issue with 25 states, new issues regarding fetal research and adoption may create problems to use of the techniques. Following the US Supreme Court's decision in 1973 legalizing abortion [*Roe v. Wade,* 410 US 13 (1973)], several states, in the name of human dignity, felt it was necessary to pass legislation banning fetal research. Defining the term fetus explicitly, the term includes not only an embryo, but any product of conception. If in vitro methods, embryo transfer and freezing and storage of embryos are interpreted as experimentation with no clear therapeutic benefit to the fetus, obstacles to the procedures may be legislated. What is construed as research varies. Some states consider fetal research as occurring only at the time of anticipated abortion or subsequent to abortion, while others consider fetal research as occurring when there is presence of fetal cardiorespiratory function, muscular activity or pulsation of umbilical vessels. In vitro fertilization falls into neither of the above categories since it neither affects abortion nor is related to issues of extra-uterine fetal function. More general laws regarding fetal research may inhibit in vitro practice if laws state that no research on a live human embryo can be performed if there is risk to its life and health.

In the matter of embryo transfer, the abortion laws may impede the procedure since removal of the fertilized ovum for transfer may be considered an abortive technique. Restraints on a woman's ova which are fertilized and transferred include prohibition on the sale of fetuses for experimentation, or for donation to others. Some states require that all the fertilized eggs be reimplanted in the same woman.

The hiring of a surrogate presents the problem of the sales of children. Many states prohibit payment to a mother for her giving up a child for adoption, thus surrogates also may not be paid. Another ruling granted the fundamental right to a couple regarding reproductive decisions which require aid from a third party – the surrogate, but that this right does not give the surrogate the right to accept pay and use adoption laws to deliver the child to the involved couple. Lawyers also may be prohibited from receiving fees for helping match surrogates with couples and placing a child for adoption.

Legal parenthood is also difficult to determine. Who are the legal parents when fertilization occurs from a third party's gamete? Most recent court rulings hold that artificial insemination of a married woman with husband consent results in a legal child of the couple. A donor is usually not considered a legal father when providing sperm for insemination of a woman to whom he is not married. This frees male donors, but can be problematic for women surrogates, if the donor decides to claim legal paternity. The female surrogate may also claim parental rights, and may want the child herself. Most laws recognize the woman who gives birth as the legal mother. A female carrier of a fertilized ovum from gametes from a husband and wife, may change her mind and wish to keep the baby. The genetic parents may have difficulty in gaining custody under the present laws. Children born with defects may be rejected by any of the parties. A decision by a surrogate to abort the pregnancy or inappropriate screening of the donor or surrogate mother for physical or psychological disorders can also result in tragedy.

The rights of and the effects on the child of in vitro insemination need to be determined. If the legal consequences are still inadequately considered, then the far-reaching psychological and emotional consequences have yet to be addressed. A research attorney notes that it is now possible for a child to have up to 5 parents: an egg donor, a sperm donor, a surrogate mother who carries the pregnancy, a couple who serve as parents. This collaboration in parenting requires better protection by current laws, better assessment of the motivation for procreation of both the couple desiring a child as well as the third parties, donors and surrogates [2].

References

1 Biggers, J.D.: In vitro fertilization and embryo transfer in human beings. New Engl. J. Med. *304:* 336–342 (1981).
2 Andrews, L.B.: The stork market: the law of the new reproductive techniques. Am. Bar. Ass. J. *70:* 50–56 (1984).

E.C. Small, MD, University of Nevada, Obstetrics and Gynecology,
School of Medicine, Reno, NV 89557 (USA)

Advances in the Diagnosis and Treatment of Chronic Pelvic Pain

Gay M. Guzinski

Division of Gynecology, University of Maryland School of Medicine and Hospital, Baltimore, Md., USA

Chronic Pain

Pain is a personal experience of an unpleasant bodily sensation. There is a 'tissue damage' or anatomic component and a reactive or emotional component to this experience. There is no standard laboratory test to measure either aspect, however, making quantification and study of pain difficult at best.

Even the most casual observer will, with a little thought, come up with examples that prove pain is more than tissue damage alone; for example, the soldier wounded in combat who needs little if any pain medication while awaiting medical evacuation away from the front line, the father who seemingly ignores serious injuries while working to free his family trapped by an accident in their car, the motorcyclist with excruciating 'phantom limb pain' following traumatic amputation of an extremity, the woman who still has monthly 'menstrual cramps' following a hysterectomy. Yet, it was only recently that the multifactorial nature of the pain experience was conceptualized. This was well stated by Dr. *John Bonica,* Chairman Emeritus and Professor, Department of Anesthesia at the University of Washington in Seattle. In 1979, he stated in a letter to the editor of the *International Journal for the Study of Pain:*

'To my mind, there is now compelling evidence that cognitive, motivational, judgemental, and psychologic processes which result from learning personality, past experience, culture and conditioning among other factors influence the transmission of nociceptive impulses at the very first synapse and at all subsequent levels along the neuraxis... consequently, [pain] cannot be artificially dichotomized into sensory pain and pain associated with emotional components' [1].

This statement emphasized that tissue damage and psychic factors far from being mutually exclusive are woven together in producing the symptom for which the patient is seeking help. The clinician's job is not, therefore, to eliminate one or the other, but rather to investigate both factors simultaneously.

The medical problems giving rise to gynecologic pain are well known to the gynecologist, and usually well evaluated. Advances are currently being made in many of these areas. Infectious diseases can cause chronic pain and current research is identifying new agents of this group of communicable disease which are causal in chronic or recurrent infectious states. Endometriosis is a problem long associated with chronic pelvic pain, and there is presently intense research on etiology and therapy for this problem. Adhesions can lead to chronic pain, and their nature and etiology is of interest to many gynecologists, most particularly those working in the field of infertility. Structural aberrations such as loss of pelvic support can be painful, but great caution is now being exercised in attributing pain solely to this problem. Tumors of the internal genitalia are remarkable for their lack of pain inspite of enormous distortion of pelvic organs. Little is known, however, of the reason for this, but it should be of research interest to gynecologic pain specialists. Nongenital structures such as the bowel, urinary tract, connective tissue and musculoskeletal system are usually considered in the differential diagnosis, and appropriate studies are undertaken to evaluate the structural contribution of these organ systems to chronic pelvic pain.

The gynecologic clinician, indeed, usually formulates an accurate assessment of how much pain should normally be produced by a degree of tissue damage that is validated by repeated experiences with acutely ill patients. Patients complaining of chronic pelvic pain, however, remain enigmatic, as the most astonishing amount of damage, for example from ovarian cancer, is often painless while very minor degrees of structural abnormality, such as adhesions, may be present in patients complaining of excruciating pain. The answer lies in the special nature of the pain experience with the ultimate complaint resulting from both the patient's physical condition and behavioral factors.

Experts in behavioral medicine have studied pain and developed new theories of describing its meaning. Pain functions as a warning of damage and a way of alerting the body to prevent further injury. This is usually clear in acute pain circumstances, but in chronic pain, the logic of the 'warning' and the nature of the further damages are obscure. In fact, chronic pain usually does not signify progressive structural damage which might, for example, lead to infertility or necessitate castration. Nor does it escalate to an unbearable level, but the fear of this is present constantly in the patient's mind and contributes to the pelvic pain patient's anxiety.

Pain is also used as a way of relating to people. The experience of pain and particularly the emitting of pain behaviors such as groaning, crying, or clutching the body all usually produce support, help, and attention in those around the patient as well as allow the patient to avoid certain activities. For example, the pelvic pain patient may receive sympathy and help at work and avoid sexual activity because of her problem. This attention may be desirable and unconscious repetition of the pain-related behavior will recur reinforced by the behavior of others.

Pain and guilt are also linked. The patient learns as a child that pain is a part of punishment when one is 'bad', so the patient who has done something she interprets as 'bad' may, as an adult, experience pain in place of feeling guilty. Pelvic pain patients may experience these feelings associated with sexual activity. The suffering endured also allows reestablishment of a good relationship with the individual doing the punishing because the price for the bad behavior has been pain. Pelvic pain patients, for example, may have sexual urges, deny a partner sexual congress, experience pain, and then feel the relationship can be 'good' again because the pain expirates the guilt from the sexuality. This entire process is usually unconscious in the patient and is generally not part of the gynecologist's concept of pain.

Finally, pain or a 'somatic symptom' may be the result of the patient's converting an unacceptable problem such as anger into an acceptable symptom such as headache, for which help can legitimately be sought. Patients who handle problems and stress in this fashion develop a whole range of somatic complaints and vigorously deny the role of contributing factors except physical illness.

Knowledge of these advances in the concepts of pain aids the health care provider in understanding and evaluating the patient presenting with chronic pain of any kind. A good review can be found in *Engel's* [2] article on psychogenic pain and the pain-prone patient in the 1959 *American Journal of Medicine*.

Chronic Pain Patients

In the recent book, *Psychological Approaches to Management of Pain*, *Victon* makes the statement that 'pain patients are especially difficult for clinicians to deal with' [3]. Advances in our understanding of why this is so have been made by many individuals.

Although most of the studies are done on patients with headaches or low back pain, the characteristics described are clearly present in patients with chronic pelvic pain. *Pilowsky* in Australia became interested in what he called illness behavior. In 1967, he reported on three primary attitudes to illness found in chronic pain patients: somatic preoccupation with disease phobia, health anxiety, and conviction of illness with nonresponse to reassurance. He and *Spence* subsequently devised a questionnaire to measure these factors in patients with chronik pain [4, 5]. Consideration of this information may help the clinician with the chronic pelvic pain patient understand the patient's resistance to psychiatric referral, as psychiatric disorders are not perceived as legitimate 'illnesses', and the pelvic pain patient's disbelief when laparoscopy fails to show sufficient organic damage to account for her pain.

Wooley [6] has commented on the fact that for chronic pain patients, the sick role has become a life-style and caretaking behaviors by medical personnel are desirable because they reinforce the validity of this role. In our society, sickness generates uncritical support and sympathy, while emotional illness does not elicit this same measure of acceptance. For this reason, gynecology patients are reluctant to exchange an organic symptom that elicits elaborate investigative attention in the medical/surgical sector and tremendous support from friends and familiy, for a psychic symptom such as depression or anxiety which may produce contempt, disgust, and criticism. The health care provider must, therefore, be careful in 'proving the patient is not sick' without considering what other roles the patient and her significant others could play and even helping them learn these new parts

Fordyce [7] has eloquently presented the operant/conditioning model for chronic pain in his book, *Behavioral Methods for Chronic Pain and Illness*. In it, he describes how patients can be conditioned to produce certain pain behaviors for the rewards they receive and how reconditioning can extinguish these undesirable traits. Although the patients described did not have chronic pelvic pain, this approach to the pain patient can be usefully applied to the patient with chronic gynecologic pain. If the office and emergency room personnel understand these patients and this approach, they can develop ways of being supportive without reinforcing the sick role by giving inappropriate medication and performing surgery which is not indicated.

Chronic pain as a variant of depressive disease has also been described by *Blumer and Heilbronn* [8] in low back pain patients. Reports of psychological testing on chronic pelvic pain patients, however, fail to report depression in all patients. Neuroticism, for example, was more commonly reported in British and European studies [9, 10].

Kolb [11] has discussed the dependency needs of chronic pain patients and described the passive dependent maneuvres these patients engage in as they attach themselves to health care providers and express anger or anxiety at detachment or separation. Indeed, pelvic pain patients frequently express hostility and indignation when the gynecologist cannot find a 'cause' for their pain, and they often imply that they are being abandoned or that the gynecologist is incompetent if the physician finds nothing sufficiently wrong with them to cause their pain. The pain patient may set the situation up for failure by initially praising the physician's competence and expressing overwhelming confidence that 'the cause will be found'. If the physician falls in with this and promises cure, the stage is set for the patient to be disappointed, depressed, and self-righteously angry when the proposed medical or surgical 'cure' has failed. Because the character of chronic pain patients has only recently come to the attention of medical personnel, chronic pelvic pain patients can find an almost unlimited number of emergence facilities, clinics, and private offices in which to enact this scene. These sadomasochistic tendencies have been well described in low back pain patients by *Blumer* [12], and should certainly be considered in the chronic pelvic pain patient.

Evaluation of Pain

The knowledge that past experience, organic damage, and current psychic functioning all contribute to the complaint of chronic pain have allowed development of a new approach to evaluation of this problem, the multidisciplinary pain clinic. In such a clinical setting, the pain sufferer is made aware at the outset that she will be taken seriously, but that her problem is complex and multifactorial, not simple and solely organic. The patient must be committed to a holistic approach to diagnosis and agree to participate in it in its entirety, rather than insist that she 'does not need' certain parts of the program. If the multidisciplinary approach is presented as providing a sophisticated, thorough evaluation of a difficult, complicated problem, patient compliance with a program can be increased. The goals of the program should be clearly outlined to the patient from the beginning as identification of the many factors contributing to the patient's pain and the development of an individualized treatment program designed to minimize these aspects. Treatment, not cure, is therefore the proposed end point, and this may require several approaches and continue for a long period of time.

The clinical program should be structured such that medical, historical, psychologic, and psychiatric data are collected, simultaneously discussed by a panel of experts, and then presented in toto at a final session with the patient. Presentation of partial results will negate the effect of the holistic approach, as the patient can insist on treatment of minor organic problems or refuse to go on with the behavioral evaluation and this 'new approach' will never have been completed. Since this approach is usually unfamiliar to the patient, the data to be discussed are extensive, and the patient's psychologic state, such as depressed or anxious, may preclude her ability to be an objective listener, she can be encouraged to bring a tape recorder or a 'significant other' to listen to the findings and recommendations.

The medical evaluation of chronic pelvic pain patients should be thorough but appropriate. Patients suspected of having an inflammatory process should have serial white cell counts and erythrocyte sedimentation rates, and appropriate cultures which might include endocervix or cul-de-sac aspirates. Laparoscopy or laparotomy may be necessary to confirm the diagnosis. If endometriosis is considered, most experts now consider visual documentation as necessary component of evaluation before any treatment plan can be formulated. Long-term antibiotic therapy should be undertaken with caution, as this medication has risk and if infection is not present, no benefit may accrue to the patient.

Structural aberrations such as pelvic relaxation or hypermobility of the uterus such as describes by *Allen and Masters* [13] may contribute to pain, but before surgical repairs alone are contemplated for pain relief, other factors should be considered. If uterine prolapse is thought to be causally related to pain, a trial of a pessary should be undertaken to determine if pain relief follows uterine elevation.

Nongenital structures such as the bowel, urinary tract, and musculoskeletal system should be investigated where appropriate. The clinician should remember that visceral sensory input is segmental and thus additive from all structures ennervated by nerves at that level. Something as simple as constipation may increase the sensory input at that level and combined with minimal tissue damage from other organs, this may exceed that patient's threshold for pain. Muscle spasms are commonly associated with chronic headache and back pain, but as *Sinaki* et al. [14] described in 1977, tension myalgia of the levators can result in suprapubic, cocygeal, rectal, sacral, and thigh pain. Palpation of the levators on rectal and vaginal exam revealed tense, firm muscle bundles that were painful, and exacerbated the patient's pain complaint. This maneuver should be part of the routine pelvic exam in patients with pelvic pain.

Of course, any masses or irregularities involving the area normally occupied by the genital organs require further investigation, possibly including intravenous urography, barium enema, and ultimately visual inspection of these structures. Laparoscopy/laparotomy should be considered in every chronic pelvic pain patient who has not had recent documentation of such findings following discussion of the risks and benefits of such a procedure. There is ample evidence that findings on physical exam are relatively poorly correlated with visible pathology, documented both by general surgeons working with trauma patients, such as *Sherwood* et al. [15], and gynecologists investigating pelvic pain like *Cunanan* et al. [16] or pelvic inflammatory disease such as *Eschenbach* [17]. The patient who has a normal pelvic exam will benefit most from having laparoscopy done in the context of the multidisciplinary plan, not to 'rule out' organic pathology. If the procedure is done alone, both the health care provider and the patient are in tacit agreement that a dichotomy between 'organic' and 'psychic' exists. Despite numerous studies in the literature including early ones such a *Castelnuevo-Tadesco and Krout* [18] in 1968 and later ones such as *Renaer* et al. [10] in 1979 describing that psychopathology was present in both patients with pelvic pathology and patients without pathology experiencing pain, the majority of gynecologists still believe that the dichotomy of organic pain and 'pain in the head' can be made. They, therefore, fail to investigate psychic factors in all patients with chronic pelvic pain and are still surprised when surgical procedures done to cure pain, when insufficient pathology is present, are failures [18]. Finally, referrals made for behavioral evaluation after the discovery that 'nothing is wrong in the pelvis' occurs are not likely to result in the patient's acceptance of this suggestion.

The behavioral aspects of pain deserve the same careful attention by experts as the medical complaints. Significant advances in pain evaluation have been made in the multidisciplinary pain centers by including social, psychologic, and psychiatric workup in the diagnostic scheme on every patient. The program administrator can often increase acceptance and compliance with behavioral evaluations by describing the contribution such common emotional states as depression and anxiety make to pain and emphasizing the reduction in pain resulting from identifying and managing those aspects of it. The implication that these problems are normal, acceptable, and treatable is reassuring rather than threatening to the pain patient.

The framework for treatment needs to be established in the diagnostic part of the patient encounter. The clinician in charge of the evaluation should validate the seriousness of the patient's complaint and attempt to determine what the patient thinks is causing the pain and what specifics she would like done about it. With this information, answers to these questions can be built into the proposed treatment plan. The goals of treatment have to include meeting the patient's dependency needs, refocusing her from a search for cure to management of her pain, and returning her to a more normal level of function.

Management of Pain

The question of appropriate treatment for chronic pelvic pain remains open. More recent thinking is that all abnormalities, even minimal ones, should be treated since it is not possible to evaluate how much they contribute to the problem of pain, moreover, thresholds for pain from small amounts of organic damage differ from patient to patient. The risks and benefits of alternative methods both medical and surgical should be carefully described, however, and the patient must decide for example whether the risks of surgery, anesthesia, and possible recurrence of the adhesions are worth the potential benefits of adhesiolysis. Gynecologists expert in pain management now recognize that surgical procedures such as hysterectomy performed solely to relieve pain in the presence of insufficient organic pathology may produce transient pain relief, but the pain usually recurs, sometimes after only a few weeks or months or relief. Current writers, most notably *Renaer* [19], concur with this and advise against this approach in nearly all cases.

Any 'trials of therapy' which are proposed should be on a clearly limited basis with reevaluation as a specified time with clear presentation of alternatives. For example, if mittelschmerz and dysmenorrhea are present and ovulation suppression is proposed, a definite number of cycles of treatment should be specified with reevaluation at that time. Even if no medically treatable condition is found, some consideration can be given to seeing the patient at set intervals, perhaps 3–4 months. This brief encounter can be used to 'determine that no new problems are developing', and maintain the therapeutic relationship thus obviating the need for the patient to 'get worse' to get an appointment. Patients often like the option of calling for brief discussion when they feel the need to talk, and it has been my experience with a large number of chronic pain patients that talking to a sympathetic nonmedical person will suffice to meet the patient's dependency needs.

The behavioral aspects of the pain need to be addressed with a simultaneous treatment program. Many options, both medical and behavioral, are available, reflecting the multifactorial nature of the problem. Medication such as antidepressants, lithium, Haldol, and other neuroleptics can be used where indicated by a confirmed psychiatric diagnosis. They should be prescribed with caution, however, and only by a practitioner trained in their use. Follow-up should be frequent, and refills of these prescriptions should again be in the hands of a psychiatric expert. In some cases, the patient can be jointly managed, and the details of follow-up will need to be worked out with the gynecologist and psychiatrist.

Other behavioral options are available. Several centers offer operant conditioning programs on an inpatient basis, and this may be appropriate for some patients. Hypnosis, biofeedback, stress management, communication skills, cognitive restructuring mediation, and small group therapy are other options which have been tried. Relaxation therapy and sexual counseling have reportedly been therapeutic [9, 20], but so has evaluation alone [21]. Nearly all reports on treatment suffer from a lack of clearly defined parameters for success, lack of controls, and short term of follow-up.

Frontiers

Given the state of our knowledge about the causes and treatment of chronic pain problems, there is room for considerable advancement in both areas. The basic science approach could yield new data in the anatomic and physiologic nature of pelvic sensation, both somatic and visceral. For example, anatomic pain pathways could be studied using horseradish peroxidase uptake and electron microscopy. Central projections of pelvic viscera might be investigated with the use of direct electrophysiologic recording from the surface of the brain. While the viscera were manipulated, laparoscopy in the awake state would allow consideration of such a study. Alteration of pelvic pain perception by hibernation state could be undertaken in those animals such as the ground squirrel where this is known to take place. Estrogen/progesterone effects on verve transmission and pain perception could be studied. The old issue of pelvic blood flow could be evaluated using laparoscopy and laser flow probes. Data corroborating *Taylor's* early studies [22] about emotional modulation of flow could even be measured in an awake patient having laparoscopy and being questioned on topics producing anger or sexual stimulation. Advances in the basic science aspects of pelvic pain are certainly needed, and technical improvements make this currently an attractive area for investigation.

Advances in treatment are clearly needed and will come from carefully designed controlled studies. Comparison of treatment programs requires that homogeneous groups of patients be placed in parallel programs with similar endpoints for success. Most published studies are noncomparable because the psychopathology and organic pathology are poorly defined so the groups are nonhomogeneous. The same treatment may be given to all patients whether or not their specific pathology indicates this. DSM III diagnoses and MMPI categorization on everyone would help with assigning these patients to specific categories so that therapies appropriate for those diagnostic categories could be developed.

Further, little attention has been paid to cultural factors in pelvic pain patients, yet symptom expression and acceptance of treatment modality may vary tremendously between even social groups. Cross-cultural studies would be of interest and would help in treatment planning. Another problem is that many studies report multiple modalities employed simultaneously, such as stress management, sexual dysfunction counselling, and supportive brief psychotherapy so that it is not possible to evaluate the effect of any single modality.

Some chronic pain treatment programs involve very sophisticated personnel interacting intensely over long periods of time with the patients. Patient compliance may be poor and the need for this long-term, complicated care by sophisticated and highly educated personnel is unproven. Perhaps trained volunteers could meet the dependency needs of these patients just as well as psychiatrists at a much lower cost. Most writers comment on the impoverished social nature of pain patients [18, 21] and their strong dependency needs [11]. Yet, little has been done on evaluating other ways of meeting those dependency needs, perhaps in an outpatient setting where 'drop-in' visits or phone calls were acceptable and handled by sympathetic personnel and frequent, brief contact was maintained with the patient. *Sternbach* [23] has pointed out that pain is a life-style. He was specifically discussing low back pain but application of this idea might provide fruitful approaches to treating pelvic pain patients. Identification of the patient's present life-style and careful delineation of what her ideal life would be like might help in structuring a treatment program desired to recondition behaviors consistent with the desired life state.

Medical approaches to chronic pelvic pain need to be further evaluated. For example, biofeedback for muscle spasm and/or pelvic congestion may prove to be useful or antidepressants could be tried in this selected chronic pelvic pain under carefully controlled, double-blind, crossover studies.

Since the goals of treatment are poorly defined, it is difficult to know what constitutes success in any one program. Advances in treatment will come only when we decide what we want to achieve and follow the patient for a long enough time to determine if that goal has been reached.

Acknowledgements

I wish to express my thanks to Dr. *John Bonica,* Dr. *Wilbert Fordyce,* and Dr. *Hans Doerr* for the privilege of working with them at the University of Washington in Seattle in the study and treatment of chronic pain.

References

1 Bonica, J.J.: Letter to the editor re: the relation of injury to pain. Pain 7: 203–207 (1979).
2 Engel, G.L.: 'Psychogenic' pain and the pain-prone patient. Am. J. Med. 26: 899–918 (1959).
3 Barber, J.; Adrian, C. (eds.): Psychological approaches to the management of pain (Brunner/Maizel, New York 1982).
4 Pilowsky, I.; Spence, N.D.: Patterns of illness behavior in patients with intractable pain. J. psychosom. Res. 19: 279–287 (1975).
5 Pilowsky, I.; Spence, N.D.: Illness behavior syndromes associated with intractable pain. Pain 2: 61–71 (1976).

6 Wooley, S.C.: Editorial proning in sick (and tired). Psychosom. Med. *42:* 233–235 (1980).
7 Fordyce, W.E.: Behavioral methods for chronic pain and illness. (Mosby, St. Louis 1976).
8 Blumer, D.; Heilbronn, M.: Chronic pain as a variant of depressive disease. The pain-prone disorder. J. nerv. ment. Dis. *1970:* 381–406 (1982).
9 Beard, W.W.; Belsey, E.M.; Liberman, B.A.; Wilkenson, J.C.M.: Pelvic pain in women. Obstet. Gynec., N.Y. *128:* 566–570 (1977).
10 Renaer, M.; Vertommen, H.; Nijs, P.; Wagemans, L.; Van Hemelrijck, T.: Psychological aspects of chronic pelvic pain in women. Am. J. Obstet. Gynec. *134:* 75–80 (1979).
11 Kolb, L.C.: Attachment behavior and pain complaints. Psychosomatics *23:* 413–425 (1982).
12 Blumer, D.: Psychiatric consideration in pain; in Rothman, Simeone, The spine (Saunders, Philadelphia 1975).
13 Allen, M.W.; Masters, W.H.: Traumatic laceration of uterine support. Am. J. Obstet. Gynec. *70:* 500–513 (1955).
14 Sinaki, M.; Merritt, J.L.; Stillwell, G.K.: Tension myalgia of the pelvic floor. Mayo Clin. Proc. *52:* 717–722 (1977).
15 Sherwood, R.; Berci, G.; Austin, E.; Morgenstern, L.: Minilaparoscopy for blunt abdominal trauma. Archs Surg., Chicago *115:* 672–673 (1980).
16 Cunanan, R.G., Jr.; Covrey, N.G.; Lippes, J.: Laparoscopic findings in patients with pelvic pain. Am. J. Obstet. Gynec. *146:* 589–591 (1983).
17 Eschenbach, D.A.: Epidemiology and diagnosis of acute pelvic inflammatory disease. Obstet. Gynec., N.Y. *55:* 1425–1535 (1980).
18 Castelnuevo-Tadesco, P.; Krout, B.M.: Psychosomatic aspects of chronic pelvic pain. Psychol. Med. *1:* 109–126 (1970).
19 Renaer, M.: Chronic pelvic pain without obvious pathology in women. Eur. J. Obstet. Gynec. *10:* 415–463 (1980).
20 Reading, A.: Chronic pain in gynecology: a psychological analysis; in Barber, Adrian, Psychological approaches to the management of pain (Brunner/Maizel, New York 1982).
21 Gross, R.J.; Doerr, H.; Caldrola, D.; Guzinski, G.; Ripley, H.S.: Borderline syndrome and incest in chronic pain patients. Int. J. Psychol. Med. *10:* 79–86 (1980/81).
22 Duncan, C.H.; Taylor, H.C.: A psychosomatic study of pelvic congestion. Am. J. Obstet. Gynec. *64:* 1–12 (1952).
23 Sternbach, R.A.: Pain patients traits and treatment (Academic Press, New York 1974).

G.M. Guzinski, MD, Division of Gynecology, University of Maryland School of Medicine and Hospital, Baltimore, MD 21201 (USA)

Sexual Dysfunctions following Diseases of the Reproductive Organs

Thomas N. Wise

Department of Psychiatry, Georgetown University Medical Center, and Department of Psychiatry, The Fairfax Hospital, Falls Church, Va., USA

The past decade has witnessed a remarkable growth of information about the role of sexuality in individuals with various medical illnesses. A published bibliography, a journal devoted to the role of sexuality and physical disability, and numerous studies now form a growing data base [1, 2]. Reproductive biology denotes sexuality. Although procreative ability is often compromised by alterations of the reproductive organs, the pleasurable and interpersonal facets of sexuality remain important in individuals despite the absence of such reproductive ability. Thus, sexual functioning in women with obstetrical and gynecological disease merits attention. This review will focus upon such conditions.

Delineation of normal psychosexual response by *Masters and Johnson* [9] allows systematic investigation of sexual dysfunctions or limitations produced by pathology in the reproductive organs. The sexual response cycle is a complex repertoire of affective, cognitive and behavioral phenomena. *Kaplan* [3] has modified the initial *Masters and Johnson* [9] description of sexual response into a tripartite cycle (see fig. 1). The initial component is a desire phase, an appetitive drive that consists of fantasies and subjective desire for sexual activity. The second phase, arousal or excitement, is characterized in the female by vaginal lubrication and progressive autonomic arousal, i. e. heart rate and rapid respiratory rate. The final phase of the sexual response cycle is that of orgasm, followed by a refractory period. The orgastic response in the normal female involves contractions within the outer third of the vaginal canal. Although far more information has been collected about male sexual response because of the peripheral anatomic nature of male tumescence, some data are available concerning the basic biology of the female psychosexual response cycle. It is

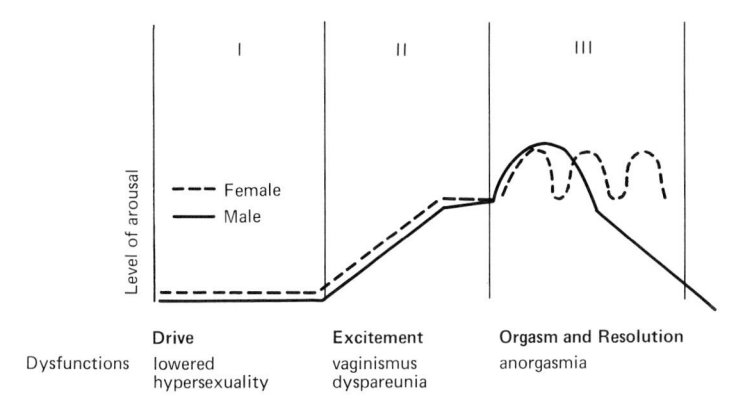

Fig. 1. Three phases of sexual dysfunction.

clear that diseases of the reproductive organs may modify such a sexual response cycle.

Biologic Basis of Sexuality

The biologic basis for sexual desire is poorly defined. Animal studies indicate that outflow tracts from the limbic system to the hypothalamus result in release of gonadotropic-releasing hormone. The pituitary-gonadal axis further modulates androgenic release. In premenopausal women, the normal cyclic variations of estrogen and progesterone apparently do not modify sexual desire. *Persky* et al. [4] were unable to document a relationship between sexual desire and estrogen and progesterone levels. *Abplanalp* et al. [5] have also questioned the cyclical nature of sexual drive in women and report only minimal psychological changes throughout the menstrual cycle. *Schreiner/Engel* et al. [6] as well as *Persky* [4] suggest a tentative relationship between androgens and adrenal cortex with sexual arousability in women. The central nervous system probably promotes sexual desire. Cortical phenomena as well as subcortical hypothalamic and preoptic areas within the brain process visual, sensory, olfactory, and gustatory sensations in addition to fantasy production that fosters sexual drive [7]. *Blumer* [8] has demonstrated that individuals, primarily male, with temporal lobe epilepsies were often hyposexual yet increase their sexual drive following drug treatment for such seizure disorders. Thus, it appears that cortical, subcortical, and endocrinologic factors modify sexual desire, although clear delineation of such physiologic phenomena is not yet available.

The next phase of the psychosexual response is the excitement phase. This appears to be mediated through the spinal cord in two centers, S2–4 and T11–12. Hemodynamic changes allow vasodilation of the pelvic genitalia. This creates a generalized swelling of the labia and tissues surrounding the vaginal barrel as well as development of the 'orgasmic platform' initially described by *Masters and Johnson* [9]. Ballooning of the inner third of the vaginal canal occurs as well. Concurrent changes also include vaginal lubrication, an exudate which is the sine qua non of the sexual excitement.

The final phase of the response cycle is that of orgasm. This consists of genital muscular contraction and involves a rhythmic contraction of the muscles around the vaginal introitus. The neurophysiology of orgasm is poorly understood, but the basic neurologic centers appear close to the anatomic centers that govern bowel and bladder functions. This is inferred from lower spinal cord injuries where orgasm as well as excretory function are ablated. *Fisher* et al. [10] recently reported a series of studies that document changes in vaginal blood flow during REM cycles. This analogous to male sexual response wherein erections occur during REM sleep, likewise vaginal blood flow develops during periods of non REM and REM sleep in a manner similar to such nocturnal penile tumescence changes.

Since *Freud's* [11] early hypothesis that there were dual orgastic responses, clitoral and vaginal, controversy persists regarding the exact phenomenology of female orgastic response. *Master and Johnson's* [9] data refute such a concept by emphasizing the unitary phenomena of orgastic release which found its base in increasing clitoral or clitoral crura stimulation that leads to this release phase of psychosexual response. A recent controversy similar to the vaginal versus clitoral orgasm is the 'G-spot controversy'. Some postulate that an area within the vaginal canal, called the Grafenberg spot, is particularly sensitive. It is also claimed that a fluid is emitted during orgasm which is analogous to the male ejaculate. A recent study conducted by *Goldberg* et al. [12] demonstrated that fluid release during orgasm comes from the urethra and may be urinary dribbling or mucus from Skene's glands. However, the documentation of a hyperesthetic spot within the vaginal canal was documented in a number of women studied, but did not correlate with orgastic response. Despite these controversies, clinical data support repeated findings that the intensity of orgasm varies from situation to situation and is not necessarily partitioned into a vaginal versus clitoral response.

Effects of Illness

Disease and distress force an individual to assume new patterns of behavior and adopt new roles because of changed responsibilities and expectations [13]. Concurrent with altered social expectations, psychological changes can set in. Illness alters human relationships and has a profound effect upon sexuality, an important medium for social interchange. The housewife suffering from ovarian carcinoma is not expected to be as good a caretaker or as good a sexual partner as when she is healthy. She is expected to seek medical aid and to get better as soon as possible. Yet, regression, reverting to old modes of behavior, can create problems for the chronically ill who will need to depend more on others but may feel uncomfortable in this role. Ignoring the psychological effects of illness and possible changes in an individual's sexual adaptation can create serious psychological problems as well as hinder medical compliance.

In considering the sexual functioning of any chronically ill person it is useful to separate out three issues [14]. First is the *psychological,* where regression and lowered self-esteem are involved. Secondly, there are the specific aspects of *organic performance* which one must consider. Individuals with physical illness have concrete reasons for altered sexual response. This can be from drugs or the technical trappings of the treatment. The individual in a full body cast will have a decreased sexual repertoire as well as the individual disfigured by severe illness that affects her reproductive organs. The specific disease state will also have marked bearing on the individual's sexual performance. The woman who undergoes a radical pelvic exenteration will have a real limitation in her 'sexual equipment'. Finally, illness can create a milieu in which the actual enjoyment is decreased although physical functioning is intact. This can be described as *organic enjoyment.* Individuals with colostomies can be worried by the fear of an order from the ostomy; individuals who have arthritis frequently find themselves in pain, as do those individuals with cord lesions who have bed sores with which to cope. Thus in considering the sexual response in women with various gynecological diseases, either acute or chronic, one must take into account the psychological, organic performance, and organic enjoyment factors. The following sections will review common gynecologic conditions where sexuality may be compromised.

Sexuality during Pregnancy and post partum

Due to major physiologic and emotional changes during pregnancy, sexuality is often affected. Psychological changes that occur depend upon the attitudes towards the pregnancy itself. If the pregnancy is desired, there will be much less ambivalence towards expectant childbirth than in unwanted pregnancy. Nevertheless, even in the most hoped for situations, ambivalent attitudes exist which can modify sexual behavior. Body image changes may create a sense of shame and disfigurement which may inhibit the individual to expose her body [15]. The attitude of the sexual partner will also determine sexual enjoyment. Disgruntled expectant fathers will diminish enjoyment of sexual relations. Sexual enjoyment may increase due to increased drive and diminished fear of conception. During gestation, sexuality is modified by the nuances of each trimester. *Masters and Johnson* [16] studied the actual physiologic changes within pregnant women. Breast engorgement seen during the first trimester may provoke heightened physical irritability and modify subjective enjoyment of breast caressing. Concurrently, during the excitement phase, multiparous women experienced dramatic labial engorgement. Increased vaginal lubrication and discharge was also noted during the first trimester. By the third trimester, the increase in vaginal engorgement obscured orgasmic contractile sensation for some subjects. During the resolution phase, the vasocongested pelvis slowly disengorged, leaving a feeling of unresolved sexual stimulation.

The subjective changes to erotic arousal vary throughout pregnancy. During the first trimester, some individuals report heightened eroticism. This was modified, however, by first trimester nausea. With the resolution of the first trimester malaise, increased sexual activity is often reported in the second trimester. Somatic complaints, such as backaches, during this period may modify sexual enjoyment [17]. Growing body changes and the tumescent abdomen may also create a sense of shame and difficulty. During the third trimester, there is a general decrease in sexual acitivity. Somatic issues such as fatigue, and difficulties in sexual position due to the turgid abdomen appear to modify the frequency of sexual activity. Utilization of side by side positions increases throughout the pregnancy.

Fear of harm to the fetus is a common inhibitor of sexual activity during the latter stages of pregnancy. In fact, there is little data to suggest that any harm occurs during intercourse. Fetal heart rate may slow slightly during orgasm in the third trimester, but a recent epidemiologic study demonstrated no relationship between fetal damage and sexual activity [18].

Immediately following delivery, sexuality is compromised by the dyspareunia and perianal pain due to tears or an episiotomy [19]. Sexuality usually returns to normal within 2 months post partum. Lactating women report erotic sensations during nursing behavior and may report losing milk during intercourse. Although sexual desire rapidly increases post partum from third trimester levels, *Tolor and Digrazio* [20] noted intercourse 7 months post partum at a lower level than prepregnancy levels in a majority of the 16 couples studied. This may relate to fatigue and preoccupation with child rearing.

In summary, sexuality during pregnancy is modified by the psychological reactions to the expected childbirth; issues of fatigue, malaise, nausea and body changes during pregnancy itself and fantasies of fetal damage. The role of the father is essential in any difficulties that do occur during this period. Fears and fantasies regarding fetal damage should be openly discussed between both sexual partners. During the postpartum period, sexuality can be compromised by fatigue, perianal pain or the vaginal dryness due to relatively low levels of estrogen following parturition.

The effect of pregnancy upon the expectant father has been succintly summarized by *Munjack and Oziel* [21]. The ambivalent feelings and expectations of the prospective father are complex and interdigitate with the pregnant mother to create a new sexual relationship. If an unplanned pregnancy forced the marriage, problems can ensue. Fears over responsibility, jealousy, issues of dependency and revivification of old parental and sibling issues all can modify sexual drive. The commitment that children entail or body image changes in the women can unconsciously stress emotionally vulnerable husbands. A clear example of the unconcious conflicts of the expectant father is found in the Couvade syndrome where the father adopts similar symptoms such as swollen abdomen, nausea, and fatigue that his pregnant wife exhibits. This unconscious identification is found frequently in modern societies in a modified form characterized by gastrointestinal symptoms indicative of regression and somatization of psychological concerns [22]. Such situations will obviously affect sexuality.

Gynecologic Surgery

Gynecologic surgery may cause various difficulties in sexual functioning. Multiple variables such as the nature of the disease, the specific treatment, the individual's support systems, and the individual's prior sexual life contribute to the specific outcome of such procedures. The hysterectomy is the most common major operation performed; almost half of these procedures include ovarian removal. The hysterectomy's effect upon sexuality should be partitioned into women who undergo the procedure for reasons other than a malignant neoplasm and those who in fact do have carcinoma or a rhabdomyosarcoma of the uterus. In women who do not have a malignancy, the psychological effects of the hysterectomy have been extensively studied. The presence of a 'posthysterectomy syndrome' has been debated but it appears that there are certain individuals who are vulnerable to such postoperative difficulties [23]. Women without any clear uterine pathology, those with a prior psychiatric illness, and women with marital difficulties appear vulnerable to such postsurgical depressive states [24, 25]. Within this setting, it is likely that sexuality may be compromised. Furthermore, these women may contribute to the common notion that sexual function following hysterectomy is often due to a barren or empty feeling. *Hunter* [26] has further clarified the matter by calling for evaluation of a 'prehysterectomy syndrome' to alert clinicians to women who are at risk.

Case 1

A 47-year-old woman was sent for psychiatric evaluation due to frequent crying spells, weight loss, and a pervasive depression. The patient stated she had undergone a hysterectomy without oophorectomy 18 months prior to consultation because of increasing menstrual blood flow and severe cramping due to uterine fibroids. Since surgery, the patient noted that she had been feeling empty and depressed. She no longer felt like a woman. The patient's past history revealed her to have been brought up in a family where religious beliefs sharply defined the role of the woman to be primarily a procreative and child-rearing member of the family. The patient had in fact raised 5 children and noted the oldest one had gone to college around the time of her surgery. Further evaluation revealed the patient to have minimal support from her husband, who was a hardworking but unsupportive individual. Difficulties with her children were also noted. Ongoing psychotherapy was recommended utilizing antidepressant medication and supportive psychotherapy.

Comment: In this woman, a tenuous homeostasis had been achieved by her functioning as a maternal figure for a large family. When the children left, increasing strains and stresses with her husband became apparent. In essence, she was a vulnerable individual and the gynecologic surgery provided a significant stress in a complex set of issues that upset her precarious balance.

Other issues may enhance sexual functioning following a hysterectomy as well as modify it. Women who are annoyed by their menstrual periods, fear pregnancy, or view their uterus only as a procreative organ, may welcome such surgery and note an improvement in their sexual relationships. *Dennerstein* et al. [27] noted that individuals with a more active sexual life tended to note improvement in their sexual response following hysterectomy, where those with a less active coital rate often noted deterioration in sexual enjoyment and sexual frequency. The actual organic changes following hysterectomy include vaginal shortening, vaginal epithelial thining, and diminished lubrication. Such anatomical changes and relative steroid starvation following oophorectomy may promote dyspareunia. Utilization of estrogen creams can reverse these changes. In some procedures part of the vaginal canal is dissected, leading to a shortened vaginal tube. Dyspareunia may thus occur in this. The absence of a cervical stump may also modify sexual enjoyment if deep penile thrusting promotes positive pelvic sensations due to cervical manipulation. Loss of the ovaries may profoundly affect sexual drive. *Zussman* et al. [28] have noted that the ovarian androgenic production may be an important source of this hormone to promote sexual drive. In its absence, libido may diminish.

Organic enjoyment factors may also compromise sexual functioning. Pelvic relaxation promotes urinary dribbling to cause urethritis or cystitis that can compromise sexual enjoyment. Weight gain and fatigue following hysterectomy, symptoms which may also be due to emotional factors, also can limit sexual enjoyment.

In summary, various factors, organic as well as psychological, modify sexual enjoyment in women with hysterectomie. The wide range of sexual difficulties following hysterectomy with or without oophorectomy from 30 to 65% make this a major concern for the physician evaluating the women about to undergo a hysterectomy. The gynecologic surgeon should asses the patient's personality, fears and fantasies about such a procedure, and be alert to any coexisting psychiatric illnesses. Follow-up care should also be directed towards investigation of sexual satisfaction and performance.

The woman who undergoes surgery for a gynecologic malignancy must be differentiated from the individuals discussed above. The meaning of such an illness will bring fear to most people. More than any other disease, the word 'cancer' brings forth fears and fantasies in both physicians and laymen [29]. The diagnosis of cancer may upset one's emotional equilibrium and impact upon one's sexual functioning independent of the treatment itself. The nuances of each particular disease must be considered. The woman with cervical carcinoma may be burdened by the additional fear that her prior sexual activities have caused this illness. Likewise, the woman with uterine cancer who has not followed up with regular gynecologic care may blame herself for her noncompliance and delay in treatment. The actual treatment itself may clearly compromise sexual activity [30–32]. Alternate forms of gratification must also be considered for the patient and her partner. The major psychological impact of a perineal exenteration will accompany the concrete loss of external genitalia. In such cases, the sexual partner should be included in support and counseling to minimize the shame as well as fear inherent in such a procedure.

Breast Disease

The breasts, although not strictly gynecological organs, are important in sexual functioning and maintenance of body image. The frequency of carcinoma of the breast and its subsequent treatment, either surgery, chemotherapy, or radiation therapy, demand investigation of the effects upon sexual functioning following treatment for carcinoma of the breast [35]. The psychological effects of such an illness may promote severe symtomatology in vulnerable individuals. *Derogatis* [36] noted that individuals who experienced depression and anxiety for 3 months following mastectomy noted significantly more sexual difficulties than those who coped without such dysphoric reactions. *Harker* [37] has noted the constant assault on one's narcissistic integrity following mastectomy. Daily viewing of the mastectomy scar and absent breast insure an ongoing reminder. *Worden and Weisman* [38] however, have demonstrated that the majority of women following mastectomy dot not have severe psychological symptoms. Thus, for most women, the anxiety and depression center around the trappings of chemotherapy following mastectomy. Nevertheless, immediately following the postoperative course, patients need the opportunity for the normal grieving process and reaccommodation to a new body image. Some individuals, however, are vulnerable to such an illness. They appear not able to cope with the narcissistic injury and change in body image.

Case 2

A 54-year-old woman was seen 6 years following mastectomy. She had been referred for persistent rage and anger towards her husband over 'looking at other women'. The patient described a very deprived, difficult childhood in a war-ravaged European country. She married an American serviceman. She prided herself on her attractiveness as the outstanding characteristic of her ability to survive her many difficulties. The patient recalled her first feelings of intense anger towards her husband while at the beach. She felt her husband was leering at other women in brief bathing suits as well as her own daughter. The narcissistic wound upon her body image and sense of self-esteem was clear throughout her ensuing psychotherapy. In the middle of psychotherapy she decided she needed a face-lift despite no ostensible reason for such a procedure. Despite multiple interpretations, she went ahead with this surgery. Although transiently relieved from her sense of depression, she rapidly relapsed into her feelings of anxiety and anger towards men, who could not have experienced 'the wound that I have incurred'.

Comment: Very narcissistic individuals with disorders of self may be vulnerable to the ravages of mastectomy.

The patient's support system, including her material stability, is an important variable in maintaining psychological health. *Jamison* et al. [39] report that those partners of mastectomy patients who had not seen their partner's naked body following surgery had less sexual satisfaction and coital orgasm than in their presurgial status. *Witkin* [40] recommends that the spouse of a mastectomy patient view the mastectomy scar in the hospital in the presence of a physician or nurse. This allows both patient and partner to view the new scar and body change in a supervised setting.

The actual biologic aspects which may limit sexual satisfaction on an organic basis appear to be related to the concrete absence of a breast, if such tactile stimulation is a major component of th individual's sexual enjoyment or their partner's, and the effects upon ovarian status following chemotherapy or radiaton treatment. Studies have noted that chemotherapeutic agents commonly used for breast cancer may impair ovarian function. This is turn may promote reduced libido as well as dryness of vaginal mucosa and result in dyspareunia [41, 42].

Finally, organic enjoyment may be impaired by soreness over the amputation, pain from swelling arms due to lymphatic blockage, and shame from other ravages of the disease. Hair loss, nausea, and vomiting from chemotherapy, pain from skeletal metastases, and general fatigue from radiation or chemotherapy or the disease process itself may all limit sexual enjoyment. Despite the above difficulties, sexual satisfaction is important in the mastectomy patient. Enhancement of self-esteem, reaffirmation of her sense of worth as a woman, and the important reality that life must go on are all important reasons for continued sexual functioning. Treatment should be directed towards areas of vulnerability. Consideration of breast protheses has also been advocated over the past few years as an approach to cope with such body image changes.

Venereal Diseases

The spectrum of venereal diseases has changed dramatically over the past century. Syphilis is now relatively uncommon, whereas gonorrhea is the most prevalent form of sexually transmitted disease. Most recently, herpes genitalis is becoming a major health problem with the dramatic rise in its prevalence. *Neisseria gonorrhoeae* infection may result in pelvic inflammatory disease and acute salpingitis [44]. Acute episodes of lower abdominal pain or chronic pelvic pain may be the sequelae of such infections. The psychological ramifications of such a disorder include shame and depression as well as anger towards the sexual partner who infected the individual. This may modify enjoyment too of any sexual activity by coupling such behavior with thoughts of the infection itself. Organic enjoyment factors include fear of infecting other individuals. The stigma of a venereal disease will also promote dysphoria. Finally, the either acute or chronic pelvic pain that results from such a disorder may cause pain upon intercourse, especially pelvic pain upon deep thrusting if chronic pelvic inflammatory disease has caused adhesions.

As herpes genitalis becomes increasingly common, the fear and shame of such an infection may limit sexual activity in the affected individual [45]. Shame of the infection promotes further distress. Individuals note that psychological stress in itself promotes recurrence of herpes infections and augments the sufferers' difficulties. These psychological difficulties as well as pain within the acute lesion will create dyspareunia at times. Ejoyment of sexuality may be limited if the individual fears further infection. Viral reactivation has also been thought to be induced by sexual intercourse. This will clearly provide a negative feedback for enjoyment of sexuality. Finally, utilization of spermatocidal foam with viridical capability has been recommended prior to intercourse. This may also upset individuals.

Treatment Considerations

In treating an individual with a disease of the reproductive organs, the role of sexuality should be considered. The individual's psychological reaction to the disease must be assessed. Specifically, the fantasies of how they developed such a disease should be elicited and any fears or disortions regarding the treatment of the condition should be considered. A woman with breast cancer who believes that her early promiscuity caused her disease may need support and information to allay that misconception. Individuals with vaginal spotting who did not seek medical care and subsequently have advanced endometrial carcinoma may suffer more then because of the knowledge that their delay in seeking treatment has severely compromised their ability to survive. The clinician should allow individuals to voice these fears and concerns. Sympathetic listening and gentle support may greatly alleviate such distressing symptoms. Actual recognition of organic limitations in sexual functioning should also be ascertained. Vaginal shortening and atrophic epithelium may promote dyspareunia. Again, the clinician's recognition that sexual activity may be the best treatment for vaginal thinning can enhance the patient's sense of self-esteem. As noted, major surgical procedures which cause body disfigurement may concretely limit sexual enjoyment but also diminish sexual enjoyment on a psychological basis due to body image changes and resultant shame. In this setting, support and discussion with both the patient and her sexual partner may enhance sexual enjoyment and activity.

Thus, utilization of a tripartite schema recognizing psychological changes secondary to an illness; concrete sexual limitations due to the illness or treatment, and areas that may limit sexual enjoyment due to pain, both physical and psychological, will allow the clinician to make a systematic assessment. These data should then be taken in the context of the individual's life. Their age, availability of sexual partners, and prior sexual attitudes and history become important in assessing the relative importance of full sexual activity. Not all individuals will view sexuality as the most important facet in their life. For the women with a major pelvic exenteration, the length of live as well as minimization of pain and suffering often far outweigh the sense of castration and disfigurement. As individuals, however, begin to recuperate, and a sense of restoration of life emerges, the role of sexuality can be important. It is often in this phase of treatment that the gynecological surgeon will be less involved. Utilization of mental health personnel with training in sexual therapy may be helpful. It is important for the clinician to attempt to utilize individuals with proper training, as too rapid or inappropriate treatment devoted to sexual therapy may cause more distress than help [46].

In summary, sexual functioning is an important medium for personal and interpersonal pleasure and communication. By recognizing its role within various gynecologic diseases, this facet of an individual's behavior can be considered and not necessarily avoided. Sexuality must be seen, however, in the full context of the patient's life and social system and not given a prioritization that resides more in the therapist's mind than in the patient.

References

1. Shaked, A.: Human sexuality in physical and mental illness and disabilities (Indiana University Press, Bloomington 1978).
2. Shaked, A.S.: Sexuality and disability (Human Sciences Press, New York 1977).
3. Kaplan, H.S.: Disorders of sexual desire, pp. 37–47, (Brunner-Mazel, New York 1979).
4. Persky, H.; Dreisbach, L.; Miller, W.R.; et al.: The relation of plasma androgen levels to sexual behaviors and attitudes of women. Psychosom. Med. *44:* 305–319 (1982).
5. Abplanalp, J.M.; Rose, R.M.; Donelly, A.F.; et al.: Psychoendocrinology of the menstrual cycle. II. The relationship between enjoyment of activities, moods, and reproductive hormones. Psychosom. Med. *41:* 605–612 (1979).
6. Schreiner-Engel, P.; Schiavi, R.C.; Smith, H.; et al.: Sexual arousability and the menstrual cycle. Psychosom Med. *43:* 199–214 (1981).
7. Robinson, R.G.: Sexual differentiation of the brain and human sexual behavior; in Meyer, Schmidt, Wise, Clinical management of sexual disorders, pp. 12–22 (Williams & Wilkins, Baltimore 1983).
8. Blumer, D.: The sexual behavior of patients with temporal lobe epilepsy before and after surgical treatment. J neuro-visc. Relat., suppl., pp. 469–476 (1971).
9. Masters, W.H.; Johnson, V.E.: Human sexual inadequacy. (Little, Brown, Boston 1970).
10. Fisher, C.; Cohen, H.D.; Schiavi, R.C.; et al.: Patterns of female sexual arousal during sleep and waking: vaginal thermoconductance studies. Archs. sex. Behav. *12:* 97–122 (1983).
11. Freud, S.: Female sexuality. Collected papers, vol. 5 (Basic, New York 1959).
12. Goldberg, D.C.; Whipple, B.; Fishkin, R.E.; et al.: The Grafenberg spot and female ejaculation. J. Sex marit. Ther. *9:* 27–37 (1983).
13. Parsons, T.: The social system, pp. 428–473 (Free Press, New York 1951).
14. Wise, T.N.: Sexuality in chronic illness. Prim. Car *4:* 199–208 (1977).
15. Perkins, R.P.: Sexuality in pregnancy: what determines behavior? Obstet. Gynec., N.Y. *59:* 189–198 (1982).
16. Masters, W.H.; Johnson, V.E.: Human sexual response, pp. 141–168 (Little, Brown, Boston 1966).
17. Reamy, K.; White, S.E.; Daniell, W.C.; et al.: Sexuality and pregnancy. J. reprod. Med. *27:* 321–327 (1982).
18. Mills, J.L.; Harlap, S.; Harley, E.E.: Should coitus late in pregnancy be discouraged? Lancet *ii:* 136–138 (1981).
19. Kerr, C.H.: Obsteric trauma and subsequent sex relations. Med. aspects hum. Sexuality *5:* 28, 40–41 (1971).
20. Tolor, A.; Digrazio, P.V.: Sexual attitudes an behavior patterns during and following pregnancy. Archs. sex. Behav. *5:* 539–547 (1976).
21. Munjack, D.J.; Oziel, L.J.: Sexual medicine and counseling in office practice, pp. 193–194 (Little, Brown, Boston 1980).
22. Trethowan, W.H.; Conlon, M.F.: The couvade syndrome. Br. J. Psychiat. *111:* 57–61 (1965).
23. Richards, D.M.: A post-hysterectomy syndrome. Lancet *ii:* 983–985 (1974).
24. Roeske, N.C.A.: Quality of live and factors affecting the response to hysterectomy. J. Fam. Prac. *7:* 483–488 (1978).

25 Polivy, J.: Psychological reactions to hysterectomy: a critical review. Am. J. Obstet. Gynec. *118:* 417–426 (1974).
26 Hunter, D.J.S.: Effects of hysterectomy. Lancet *ii:* 1265–1266 (1974).
27 Dennerstein, L.; Wood, C.; Burrows, G.D.: Sexual response following hysterectomy and oophorectomy. Obstet. Gynec., N.Y. *49:* 9–96 (1977).
28 Zussmann, L.; Zussmann, S.; Sunley, R.; et al.: Sexual response after hysterectomy-oophorectomy. Am. J. Obstet. Gynec. *140:* 725–730 (1981).
29 Wyler. A.R.; Masuda, M.; Holmes, T.H.: Seriousness of illness rating scale. J. psychosom. Res. *14:* 59–64 (1969).
30 Vicent, C.E.; Vicent, B.; Greiss, F.C.; et al.: Some marital-sexual concomitants of carcinoma of the cervix. Southern Med. J. *68:* 552–558 (1975).
31 Decker, W.H.; Schwartzmann, E.: Sexual function following treatment of carcinoma of the cervix. Am. J. Obstet. Gynec. *83:* 401–405 (1962).
32 Seibel, M.M; Freeman, M.G.; Graves, W.L.: Carcinoma of the cervix and sexual function. Obstet. Gynec., N.Y. *55:* 484–487 (1980).
33 Brown, R.S.; Haddox, V.; Posada, A.; et al.: Social and psychological adjustment following pelvic exenteration. Am. J. Obstet. Gynec. *114:* 162–171 (1972).
34 Morley, G.W.; Lindenauer, S. M.; Youngs, D.D.: Vaginal reconstruction following pelvic exenteration. Am. J. Obstet. Gynec. *116:* 996–1002 (1973).
35 Bransfield, D.D.: Breast cancer and sexual functioning: a review of the literature and implications for future research. Int. J. Psych. Med. *12:* 197–211 (1982).
36 Derogatis, L.R.: Breast cancer and gynecologic cancer – their unique impact on body image and sexual identity in women. Front. Radiat. Ther. Onc., vol. 141 1–11 (Karger, Basel 1980).
37 Harker, B.L.: Cancer and communication problems; a personal experience. Int. J. Psych. Med. *3:* 163–171 (1972).
38 Worden, J.W.; Weisman, A.D.: The fallacy in postmastectomy depression. Am. J. med. Sci. *273:* 169–175 (1977).
39 Jamison, K.R.; Wellison, D. K.; Pasnau, R.O: Psychosocial aspects of mastectomy. I. The women's perspective. Am. J. Psychiat. *135:* 432–436 (1978).
40 Witkin, M.H.: Psychosexual counseling of the mastectomy patient. J. Sex marit. Ther. *4:* 30–28 (1978).
41 Seiber, S.M.; Adamson, R.H.: Toxicity of antineoplastics in man: chromosomal aberrations, antifertility effects, congenital malformation and carcinogenic potential. Adv. Cancer Res. *22:* 57–155 (1975).
42 Yancey, R.C.: Complications of cancer chemotherapy. Cancer Bull. *32:* 11–22 (1980).
43 Schain, W.S.: Sexual functioning, self-esteem and cancer care. Front. Radiat. Ther. Onc., vol. 14 12–19 (1980).
44 Potterat, J.J.; Phillips, L.; Rothenberg, R.B.; et al.: Gonococcal pelvic inflammatory disease. Am. J. Obstet. Gynec. *138:* 1101–1104 (1980).
45 Herpes Resource Center: Psychological responses to genital herpes. Helper *3:* 2–3 (1981).
46 Meyer, J.K.: Training and accreditation for the treatment of sexual disorders. Am. J. Psychiat. *133:* 389 (1976).

Thomas N. Wise, MD, Georgetown University Medical Center, Chairman, Department of Psychiatry, The Fairfax Hospital, Falls Church, VA 22046 (USA)

Use of Behavior Therapy in Obstetrics and Gynecology

Elizabeth A. Klonoff[a], Jeffrey W. Janata[b]

[a] Departments of Psychiatry, Pediatrics, and Neurology, and [b] Department of Psychiatry, Case Western Reserve University, Cleveland, Ohio, USA

Recently, both the medical and the psychological literature have shown a dramatic increase in the use of psychological techniques to treat physically based problems. In general, a wide array of physical systems and medical specialities have been represented. In many instances, the approach taken reflects a behavior therapy orientation [e. g., *Doleys* et al., 1982]. Despite a significant amount of work in such areas as smoking cessation [*Lichtenstein,* 1982], headache [*Blanchard and Andrassik,* 1982], gastrointestinal disorders [*Whitehead and Bosmajian,* 1982], arthritis [*Achterberg-Lawlis,* 1982], and diabetes [*Fisher* et al., 1982], relatively little has been written about the use of behavioral techniques in the area of obstetrics and gynecology. The purpose of the current paper is to review the available literature in this area. First, commonly used behavioral interventions will be described. Second, where a body of literature relevant to the management of an obstetric or gynecologic patient has already been developed, its applicability to this population will be noted. And third, areas which merit additional research will be described.

For purposes of the current paper, the field of obstetrics and gynecology will be divided into five major areas. Specifically, these include: (1) problems associated with menstruation, including both dysmenorrhea and premenstrual syndrome; (2) pregnancy and delivery, including both difficulties due to the pregnancy itself and problems resulting from reluctance to prescribe medications to the pregnant woman; (3) gynecologic pain, including vaginismus, dyspareunia, and chronic pelvic pain; (4) issues related to menopause, and (5) problems related the treatment and management of the patient with gynecologic cancer. Behavioral approaches to specific sexual dysfunctions (e. g., inorgasmic dysfunction) will not be covered in the current review, as there are many reviews of such approaches in this area [e. g., *Walker*, 1982].

Common Behavioral Interventions

The experimental literature contains a number of empirically demonstrated behavioral techniques. In addition, a number of comprehensive summaries of the use of behavior therapy are available. Some of these are problem-focused, where the interventions used to treat a specific problem are reviewed [e. g. *Turner* et al., 1981]; others are intervention-focused, where the theoretical basis of the intervention is the major organizing strategy [e. g. *Rimm and Masters*, 1979]. Because assessment is such an integral part of the behavioral approach, a number of books devoted to behavioral assessment of adult [e. g., *Hersen and Bellack*, 1981] and child [*Ollendick and Hersen*, 1984] problems may also be found. A complete review of the array of behavioral interventions is beyond the scope of this article; thus, we will describe the behavioral interventions most often utilized for psychophysiological or medical problems.

Operant Conditioning

Operant conditioning reflects the stereotype most people have about behavior therapy approaches. In essence, operant conditioning focuses on two aspects of the patient's behavior: the antecedents, or events preceding or associated with the occurrence of the behavior; and consequences, or events that either immediately follow or are viewed by the patient as being the result of the behavior. Thus, operant conditioning looks at whether behavior is reinforced (rewarded) or punished. Situations in which the individual is likely to experience the problem are assessed and attempts are made to teach an alternative response. In essence, the operant conditioning model asks to what degree a medical problem or symptom presentation represents a learned behavior on the part of the patient.

A number of clinical implications derive directly from the operant conditioning model. For example, the attention and concern of a warm supportive physician and his/her staff may, in some instances, serve to reinforce or maintain the patient's symptom complaints. This is more likely in chronic conditions than in acute illnesses. The operant model would suggest that reversing the reinforcers, that is, paying attention to the patient when she is feeling better rather than only when she is feeling worse, may significantly decrease the likelihood of repeated complaints. This approach has been used with a wide variety of medical problems including astasia-abasia [e.g. *Janata and Klonoff,* 1983], chronic pain [e.g. *Fordyce,* 1976], chronic factitious illness [*Klonoff* et al., 1983], and repeated respiratory arrest [*Janata and Klonoff,* 1983].

Systematic Desensitization

First developed by *Wolpe* [1958], this approach is widely used in treatment of problems associated with fear and axiety. Classic systematic desensitization consists of three major components. First, the patient's approach to the feared object is broken down into a number (typically 15 or 20) of small steps. The approach is conceptualized along either a spatial/ temporal (e.g. how long or how far the feared event is from the patient) or conceptual (e.g. how much of the event the patient can tolerate) basis. Once identified, these steps are then sequenced in hierarchical order from least anxiety-invoking to the most stressful step the patient could imagine. Development of the hierarchy is the first step necessary for systematic desensitization. Concurrent with the hierarchy development, the patient is taught relaxation techniques. Typically, these techniques involve progressive relaxation [*Jacobson,* 1938]; recently, other inductions such as autogenic training [*Schultz and Luthe,* 1959] or the *Benson* [1975] procedure have also been used. Learning to relax, then, a response that is incompatible with anxiety, is the second major component. The third consists of having the patient imagine each step in the hierarchy while maintaining a state of relaxation. Pairing the image of the feared item with a state of relaxation makes the patient more comfortable with the actual situation when it is later encountered. If the patient experiences discomfort during the pairing process, she is instructed to stop imagining and return to relaxing. Thus, systematic desensitization is, by design, relatively anxiety-free. Although originally conceptualized as a totally imaginary process, recent innovations include applying the general paradigm to in vivo situations. In those cases, the patient actually puts herself in the feared situation while attempting to remain relaxed.

Although systematic desensitization per se is not used often in medical practice, a number of general principles have been extracted and comprised major components of the behavioral treatment of psychophysiologic problems. Specifically, these aspects include: breaking the problem down into small component steps; using relaxation as a method of coping with stress; moving the patient systematically and slowly through graduated steps towards increased health and keeping anxiety to a minimum. Many of these principles are applicable to a variety of conditions.

Biofeedback

Biofeedback represents a relatively new clinical technique that has gained much attention recently. A number of recent books [*Olten and Noonberg,* 1980] and professional journals *(Biofeedback and Self-Regulation)* reflect this increased interest. Biofeedback represents a melding of improved ability to measure physiological response and increased knowledge regarding how people learn best. Minute changes in physiologic response (typically surface electromyographic response or digital temperature) are measured and information about these changes are 'fed back' to the patient through either a variable auditory tone or light display. In this way, a patient can learn to bring these physiological responses under volitional control.

Although initially viewed as a potential cure for all psychophysiological problems, recent reviews suggest that the actual success of biofeedback techniques is significantly more limited. *Tarler-Benlolo* [1978], in a review of biofeedback treatment of pain, concluded that these techniques may not be significantly better than the simple induction of relaxation. Other investigators provide evidence of specific benefits of biofeedback [*Andrasik* et al., 1982]. From a psychological perspective, biofeedback may be useful because it can serve as a conceptual bridge for the patient with a psychophysiologic disorder [*Klonoff* et al., 1983]. Because of its physiologic basis, patients with psychologically mediated medical problems may accept biofeedback more readily than traditional psychiatric treatment. Once a patient enters into treatment, psychologic issues can then be addressed from the perspective of stress and its impact on the patient. Thus, the use of biofeedback may be one method of treating patients who would otherwise refuse psychologic or psychiatric intervention.

Cognitive Techniques

Recently, the behavioral literature has expanded to include interventions reflecting a more cognitively oriented approach. Cognitive behavior therapy contends that it is a patient's reaction to a situation, not specific reinforcers or punishers in the situation, that cause increased stress. It emphasizes teaching patients to recognize irrational beliefs, to evaluate the degree to which those irrational beliefs affect their lives, and to slowly and systematically change those irrational beliefs with the therapist's assistance.

These irrational beliefs include such statements as 'I must be perfect in everything I do' or 'Everyone must love me all the time' [borrowed from *Ellis,* 1962]. The introduction of cognition into behavioral approaches represents a significant step, as it increases the likelihood of rapprochement with more traditional orientations and broadens the scope of behavioral interventions. The cognitive approach has been particularly useful in assisting people to cope with or manage life stress. Because stress is often cited as an underlying component of psychophysiologic problems, cognitive approaches are particularly relevant in the treatment of medical problems.

Problems Associated with Menstruation

Both the laypress and the professional community have recently devoted significant attention to the problem of premenstrual syndrome. Premenstrual syndrome is associated with certain physiologic and affectional changes commensurate with, or immediately preceding, the time of menstruation. In general, much of the work has focused on attempts to document the existence of the syndrome [e. g. *Ruble,* 1977] or attempts to treat the problem utilizing hormonal therapies. However, well-controlled clinical treatment studies utilizing clear objective criteria for the diagnosis of premenstrual syndrome are still lacking.

A number of symptoms associated with premenstrual syndrome have been demonstrated to be affected, at least in part, by behavioral techniques. Primary among these is the problem of dysmenorrhea. *Mullen* [1968] described the treatment of a 31-year-old woman who had suffered from dysmenorrhea for 21 years. Treatment consisted primarily of systematic desensitization, relaxation training, and a re-learning procedure. Many of the hierarchy items used during desensitization were related to menstruation. *Mullen* [1971] replicated this successful use of systematic desensitization with an additional 5 college women. When compared, significant differences were found pre- und post-treatment on the symptom rating scale.

Tasto and Chesney [1974] treated 7 students utilizing group muscle relaxation training and imagery regarding pain reduction during menstruation. Small groups of subjects met for 5 sessions over a period of 4 weeks. All subjects reported significant benefit from this approach. However, in a later article [*Chesney and Tasto,* 1975] they suggest that behavior therapy and muscle relaxation might be more effective in spasmodic rather than congestive dysmenorrhea. 69 volunteers were assigned to one of six groups in a 2 (congestive vs. spasmodic) by 3 (behavior therapy vs. pseudotreatment vs. waiting list) factorial design. Although clearly limited in terms of sample generalization, their results were interpreted to suggest that behavioral approaches may be effective in reducing the symptomatology of spasmodic dysmenorrhea but not congestive dysmenorrhea.

In addition to generalized relaxation training, biofeedback has also been used to treat problems associated with menstrual pain. Although somewhat anecdotal in nature, these results suggest potentially positive treatment effects. For example, *Adler and Adler* [1979] reported 5 patients receiving temperature feedback for migraine headaches who spontaneously noted the disappearance of dysmenorrhea symptoms. *Tubbs and Carnahan* [1976] reported on 10 subjects woh received both EMG and temperature biofeedback; of these, 4 showed dramatic, while 2 showed moderate improvement. *Dietvoise and Osborne* [1978] reported positive effects in a patient who had not responded to hormone therapy and analgesics. *Heczey* [1977] utilized autogenic relaxation and vaginal temperature feedback with 44 college women. The women were divided into four groups including: no training control, group autogenic training, individual autogenic training, and relaxation and vaginal temperature feedback. Improvement rate for those individuals who received autogenic training and biofeedback was 92%, while improvement for individual and group autogenic training was 76 and 64%, respectively. This suggests that, at least for some forms of dysmenorrhea, behavior therapy and some form of relaxation therapy may be useful.

Another aspect of premenstrual symptom often mentioned is change in affect. Two changes are typically described, increased depression and increased anger outbursts. Treatment of both of these problems has been described in the behavioral literature. Research evidence has demonstrated the efficacy of a cognitive behavioral approach in the treatment of depression [*Beck*, 1967]. In some respects, this represents a change in attribution, the way the patient explains what is going on around her. To date, this systematic changing of attributions has not been experimentally evaluated in women experiencing premenstrual depression. In addition, many women will report significantly more anger outbursts during this time. Protocols for helping patients to cope with feelings of out-of-control anger have been developed [e. g., *Novaco*, 1977]. Again, to our knowledge, these protocols have not been systematically applied to women with identified premenstrual anger problems. Once the problem of adequate definition of those women with premenstrual syndrome is solved, a number of research areas for the behaviorally oriented practitioner are available. Even without the clear identification of a 'syndrome', many of the symptoms women experience at the time of menstruation may be alleviated through behavioral approaches.

Problems Associated with Pregnancy

For some time psychological factors have been thought to influence both the course of pregnancy and the process of childbirth. *McDonald* [1968] reviewed studies which examined obstetric complications in light of emotional factors, which factors he concluded consistently differentiated normal and complication samples. In particular, self-reported anxiety seemed to be the most potent psychological factor differentiating complicated from uncomplicated pregnancies. *Gorsuch and Key* [1974] examined the roles of state anxiety and stress in medical abnormalities in pregnancy. Studying the course of pregnancy in 118 women, these researchers found an independent and significant influence of both anxiety and life stress. State anxiety during the first trimester, and the occurrence of life changes and stress during the second and third trimesters were positively correlated with both the presence of and number of pregnancy abnormalities. The efficacy of behavioral management of state anxiety and stress is well established, yet to our knowledge the effect of these techniques on pregnancy complications has not been systematically studied.

Anxiety has also been thought to be a major factor in labor pain and delivery complications [e. g. *Astbury,* 1980]. Relaxation for control of pain and anxiety during labor has been featured prominently in most current prenatal education programs. Most women consider this type of training to be helpful and there is evidence that prophylactic childbirth training is effective in reducing pain, but that the degree to which pain is reduced is not as great as is generally believed [*Melzack* et al., 1981]. Several researchers have employed biofeedback-assisted relaxation training as a component of prenatal training. *Gregg* [1978] noted a reduction in the amount of analgesic medications used and briefer first stage labor in a group of patients trained using biofeedback. *St. James-Roberts* et al. [1982, 1983] criticized this research as being less than adequately controlled and having included substantial amounts of additional psychological preparation, masking the biofeedback-specific effects. These researchers, apparently reporting the same study twice, compared electromyographic and skin conductance biofeedback training effects on labor and delivery. Based on self-report and postnatal interviews, they concluded that the biofeedback apparati were useful in aiding relaxation and providing distraction during early labor, but that with more frequent contractions relaxation proved to not be significantly useful.

Behavioral pain management approaches seem particularly useful during the course of pregnancy to treat pain whose pharmacologic management is contraindicated. For example, tricyclic antidepressants are often used to treat migraine headache, but have not been established as safe during pregnancy and lactation. Similarly, there are a variety of chronic and acute pain conditions for which medications are the standard treatment, but a quick perusal of the PDR demonstrated that a number of these medications are not judged safe for pregnant or lactating women. Our experience has been that behavioral pain management techniques are an effective alternative.

Problems Associated with Pain

Vaginismus and Dyspareunia

The systematic treatment of problems associated with vaginismus has been previously reported [*Lamont, 1978*]. In general, this approach is a variant of systematic desensitization. The patient is instructed to use increasingly larger vaginal dilators until she is able to comfortably and without anxiety regain some control over the introital muscles. As with systematic desensitization, the patient is encouraged to not move to the next dilator size until she feels she can successfully and comfortably accommodate the size she is currently using. Although many patients (and, unfortunately, many practitioners) interpret *Lamont's* recommendations to be 'stretching' the vagina, that conceptualization ignores the anxiety and other psychological factors that may be contributory. Experience using desensitization suggests that maintaining a high level of comfort for the patient and returning a sense of control are critically important to successfully deconditioning the classically conditioned tightening response associated with the sensation of something entering the vagina.

In general, the treatment of dyspareunia followed the same approach. Both organic cause and a more specific sexual dysfunction (such as inorgasmic dysfunction that mitigates adequate lubrication of the vagina) must first be ruled out. Following this, treatment is done in much the same way as *Lamont's* recommendation for vaginismus. Specifically, this involves gradually increasing both the duration and the depth of penetration during intromission while maintaining a state of cognitive relaxation. Again, as in other behavioral treatments, the important psychological component is returning a sense of control to the woman. Thus, both partners need to be seen in order to facilitate this. For a more thorough review of the treatment of dyspareunia, see *Lopiccolo and Lopiccolo* [1978].

Treatment of Chronic Pelvic Pain

Perhaps one of the most thoroughly established and researched interfaces between behavior therapy and medicine is the treatment of chronic pain [*Brena and Chapman,* 1983; *Zlutnick and Taylor,* 1982]. Specifically, the use of operant, relaxation-based, and cognitive approaches in pain management have been well established. An array of chronic pain conditions have been treated using these approaches including pain associated with carcinoma. To date, little systematic work has been reported on the behavioral treatment of chronic pelvic pain. However, it is reasonable to expect that treatment would be quite similar. As with all chronic pain conditions, the spouse needs to be actively involved in treatment, for he may be unknowingly reinforcing aspects of the pain problem. In addition, a thorough assessment of the role of pain in the patient's everyday life needs to be completed. Examples of such assessments are available [e. g. *Turk* et al., 1983]. As with all chronic pain, it may be reinforced by enabling the woman to avoid uncomfortable or unpleasant situations (e. g. divorce, housework). A possible sexual dysfunction that makes avoiding intercourse desirable must also be evaluated.

Our experience with chronic pain conditions suggests that the onset of the pain is usually associated with the actual trauma, perceived or actual tissue damage, or the onset or cessation of a major life stressor. Thus chronic pain begins as real pain; however, for some reason the experience of pain continues long after demonstrable pathology can be found. Consequently, it may be useful to employ a variant of *Lamont's* [1978] technique described above. Because chronic pain is usually experienced as uncontrollable, returning a sense of self-control over gynecologic organs may be important. In addition, marital therapy designed to help the couple cope with the problems of chronic pelvic pain needs to be included. Thus, chronic pelvic pain is another example of a problem where models for treatment from a behavioral perspective have been developed, but not systematically applied. Further research in this area should be devoted to more complete experimental trials of a comprehensive 'pain center' approach to this gynecologic problem, without resorting to additional surgeries that may only serve to exacerbate the pain condition.

Problem of Menopause

Studies have demonstrated that a high proportion of menopausal women experience troublesome symptoms, particularly hot flashes [*Polit and LaRocco,* 1980; *Thompson* et al., 1973]. Traditional treatment approaches have emphasized the use of estrogen replacement and non-hormonal medications [*Clayden* et al., 1974; *Lightman and Jacobs,* 1979], tranquilization [*Torman,* 1968], and education and reassurance [*Nonal* et al., 1975]. Each of these approaches has its limitations. Estrogen replacement has been criticized on the grounds that hormonal levels fail to adequately correlate with menopausal symptoms [*Aksel* et al., 1976], and the use of hormonal replacement has been linked with increased likelihood of cervical carcinoma [cf. *Voda,* 1981] and other potentially harmful side effects.

Recently, researchers in the field have begun to examine behavioral approaches to hot flashes. Several lines of evidence have suggested the potential efficacy of behavioral treatments.

Hot flashes and other menopausal symptoms have long been thought to correlate with stress and anxiety. *Winokur* [1973] found that 75% of his sample of menopausal women reported 'nervousness', while *Polit and Larocco* [1980] noted that 42% of the sample complained of anxiety, and a common anecdotal observation is that with increased stress and anxiety come increased frequency and severity of symptoms. This apparent relationship between stress and anxiety and menopausal symptoms suggests that the behavioral techniques used with demonstrated effectiveness to counteract anxiety and stress [cf. *Hare and Lewis,* 1981] might well be useful in the amelioration of menopausal symptoms.

Another indication of the potential usefulness of behavioral techniques is the temperature change that accompanies hot flashes. *Molnar* [1975] measured body temperature changes at several skin sites as well as monitoring core temperature. He noted that internal temperature decreases, while skin temperature at the cheek and toe increase (mean of 0.7 °C) during a hot flash. *Meldrum* et al. [1979] reported digital temperature increases averaging 2.7 °C, suggesting accompanying peripheral vasodilation. The biofeedback literature has demonstrated that significant voluntary control of skin temperature is possible, to the extent that biofeedback now seems to be the treatment of choice for Raynaud's disease [*Gugliemi* et al., 1982]. Biofeedback-based temperature control training seems a promising direction for hot flashes treatment research.

We are currently investigating the role of physical self-perception and emotional factors in the experience of hot flashes. Ambulatory monitoring of skin temperature and subject report of occurrence, duration, and intensity of hot flashes are being utilized to examine the relationship between the physiologic markers of flash activity and women's experience of hot flashes. The possible roles of anxiety, depression, and stress are being examined through the use of psychological instruments, as well as laboratory analogs of physical stress (being seated in a hot room) and psychological stress (imagining fear-producing scenes). Confirmation of relationships between these psychologic and emotional states may help lay the foundation for a comprehensive and effective behavioral treatment approach for hot flashes.

A preliminary example of the application of behavioral techniques is a study by *Stevenson and Delprato* [1983] in which women complaining of hot flashes were trained in several stress and temperature control techniques, which included relaxation, self-suggestion of cool thoughts and images, marital contingency contracting, and temperature biofeedback. Although the study was small in scale (n = 4), the results are encouraging. The mean percentage reduction in number of hot flashes between baseline and the end of training was 70%, with treatment gains maintained at 6-month follow-up. The study is limited by the inclusion of a variety of treatment strategies, which masks the relative effectiveness of each. However, the data are promising and suggest that further exploration of the use of behavioral techniques is justified.

Management of the Patient with Cancer

One relatively recent innovation in the behavioral treatment literature has been work with cancer patients. Approximately 25% of all chemotherapy patients develop aversion reactions to treatment. Typically, this takes the form of anticipatory nausea/emesis. Although more thorough reviews are available [*Redd and Andrykowski*, 1982], we will attempt to briefly describe the nonpharmacological treatments being used.

Anticipatory nausea/emesis has been conceptualized as the result of respondent, or classical conditioning [*Redd and Andresen*, 1981]. Through repeated association with chemotherapy and its negative after-effects, previously neutral events (such a coming to the hospital, the sight of the treatment room, and so forth) acquire nausea/emesis-eliciting properties. This reaction may be cognitively mediated also, with some patients becoming nauseated merely thinking about chemotherapy.

To date, four different intervention strategies have been evaluated. *Redd* et al. [1982] used therapist-directed muscle-relaxation hypnosis and guided imagery. Decreases in nausea prior to and during chemotherapy were reported by all patients when hypnosis and imagery were used. In addition, anticipatory emesis was also eliminated. However, one major problem with this approach is the apparent need for the therapist to be present with the patient for the treatment effects to occur.

Progressive muscle relaxation and guided imagery have been used in a series of studies [*Burish and Lyles,* 1979, 1981; *Lyles* et al., 1982]. A variety of physiological, observational, and self-report measures were used. These procedures produced reductions in pulse rate and blood pressure as well as reported anxiety and nausea, while patients in control conditions did not demonstrate these reductions. Again, however, problems emerged at follow-up. When the therapist was no longer with the patient, treatment benefits were dramatically reduced.

The use of multi-site EMG biofeedback and imagery has also been reported [*Burish* et al., 1981]. These results replicated earlier findings by *Burish* in that distress and nausea were reduced. In addition, systematic desensitization has also been used with similar success.

In summary, studies of relaxation-based interventions have consistently demonstrated success in reducing anticipatory nausea/emesis. However, a number of problems remain. Primary among these is the apparent need for the therapist to be present during the chemotherapy treatment for positive effects to be obtained. This is particularly costly in terms of therapist time. Second is the potential role distraction may play. Positive results may reflect less the direct benefits of relaxation and more that the procedure distracts the patient's attention from the aversive stimuli. And finally, the exact mechanism through which these interventions are effective has not been identified. As a result, it is difficult to ascertain which intervention would work best with which patient. However, results such as these suggest that, where anticipatory nausea/emesis is a problem, methods for helping patients cope are available. Additional research needs to be directed towards further refining and developing these techniques.

Conclusions

In summary, a wide variety of behavioral interventions have been shown to be effective with psychophysiological disorders. The direct applicability of these interventions to problems in obstetrics and gynecology has received relatively less attention. However, there is no reason to believe that similar successes could not be achieved with this population.

Behavior therapy represents a relatively recent, practical approach to the patient with psychophysiological disease. Many of the underlying principles, such as reinforcement and systematic desensitization, could easily be incorporated into routine office practice. Patients who are complaisant with therapeutic regimens, for example, could be given more physician attention. Giving a woman a greater sense of control during a pelvic exam by allowing her to dictate the pace and apprising her of each step before it is done is yet another example. Conceptualizing and breaking down anxiety-producing procedures into smaller steps that a woman can comfortably go through could also be done with relatively little additional effort. When the problem reaches the point where a different kind of intervention is called for, behavior therapy offers an alternative to traditional psychiatric consultation. Future research should be directed towards the systematic investigation of the use of behavioral interventions in women with obstetrical and gynecological problems.

References

Achterberg-Lawlis, J.: The psychological dimensions of arthritis. J. consult. clin. Psychol. *50:* 984–992 (1982).

Adler, C.S.; Adler, S.M.: Biofeedback and psychosomatic disorders; in Basmajian, Biofeedback: principles and practice for clinicians (Williams & Wilkins, Baltimore 1979).

Aksel, S.L.; Schonberg, D.W.; Tyrey, L.: Vasomotor symptoms, serving estrogens, and gonadotropin levels in surgical menopause. Am. J. Obstet. Gynec. *126:* 165–170 (1976).

Andrasik, F.; Coleman, D.; Epstein, L.H.: Biofeedback: clinical and research consideration; in Doleys, Meredith, Ciminero, Behavioral medicine: assessment and treatment strategies (Plenum Press, New York 1982).

Astbury, J.: The crisis of childbirth: can information and childbirth education help? J. psychosom. Res. *24:* 9 (1980).

Beck, A. T.: Depression: causes and treatment (University of Pennsylvania Press, Philadelphia 1967).

Benson, H.: The relaxation response (Morrow, New York 1975).

Blanchard, E.B.; Andrasik, F.: Psychological assessment and treatment of headache: recent developments and emerging issues. J. consult. clin. Psychol. *50:* 859–879 (1982).

Brena, S.F.; Chapman, S.L.: Management of patients with chronic pain (Spectrum, Jamaica 1983).
Burish, T.G.; Lyles, J.N.: Effectiveness of relaxation training in reducing the aversiveness of chemotherapy in the treatment of cancer. J. Behav. Ther. exp. Psychiat. *10:* 357–361 (1979).
Burish, T.G.; Lyles, J.N.: Effectiveness of relaxation training in reducing adverse reactions to cancer chemotherapy. J. behav. Med. *4:* 65–78 (1981).
Burish, T.G.; Shartner, C.D.; Lyles, J.N.: Effectiveness of multiple muscle-site EMG biofeedback and relaxation training in reducing the aversiveness of cancer chemotherapy. Biofeedback Self-Regul. *6:* 523–535 (1981).
Chesney, H.A.; Tasto, D.L.: The effectiveness of behavior modification and spasmodic and cognitive dysmenorrhoea. Behav. Res. Therapy *13:* 240–253 (1975).
Clayden, J.R.; Bell, J.W.; Pollard, P.: Menopausal flushing: double-blind trial of a non-hormonal medication. Br. med. J. *i:* 409–412 (1974).
Dietvoise, T.E.; Osborne, D.: Biofeedback-assisted relaxation training for primary dysmenorrhoea: a case study. Biofeedback Self-Regul. *3:* 301–305 (1978).
Doleys, D.M.; Meredith, R.L.; Ciminero, A.R.: Behavioral medicine: assessment and treatment strategies (Plenum Press, New York 1982).
Ellis, A.: Reason and emotion in psychotherapy (Lyle Stuart, New York 1962).
Fisher, E.B., Jr.; Delamater, A.M.; Bertelson, A.D.; Kirkley, B.G.: Pychological factors in diabetes and its treatment. J. consult. clin. Psychol. *50:* 993–1003 (1982).
Fordyce, W.E.: Behavioral methods for chronic pain and illness (Mosby, St. Louis 1976).
Gorsuch, R.L.; Key, M.K.: Abnormalities of pregnancy as a function of anxiety and life stress. Psychosom. Med. *36:* 352–363 (1974).
Gregg, R.H.: Biofeedback relaxation training effects in childbirth. Behav. Engineering *4:* 57 (1978).
Gugliemi, R.S.; Roberts, A.H.; Patterson, R.: Skin temperature biofeedback for Raynaud's disease: a double-blind study. Biofeedback Self-Regul. *7:* 99–106 (1982).
Hare, N.; Lewis, D.J.: Pervasive ('free-floating') anxiety: a search for a cause and treatment approach; in Turner, Calhoun, Adams, Handbook of clinical behavior therapy (Wiley, New York 1981).
Heczey, M.D.: Effects of biofeedback and autogenic training on menstrual experiences, relationships among anxiety, locus on control and dymenorrhoea; unpubl. PhD diss. City University of New York (1977).
Hersen, M.; Bellack, A.S.: Behavioral assessment; 2nd ed. (Pergamon Press, New York 1981).
Jacobsen, E.: Progressive relaxation (University of Chicago Press, Chicago 1938).
Janata, J.W.; Klonoff, E.A.: Behavioral treatment of repeated respiratory arrest in a pediatric patient. Annu. Meet. Ass. Advancement Behav. Ther., Washington, D.C., 1983.
Janata, J.W.; Klonoff, E.A.: Behavioral management of a case of astasia-abasia. Annu. Meet. Ass. Advancement Behav. Ther., Washington, D.C., 1983.
Klonoff, E.A.; Youngner, S.J.; Moore, D.J.; Hershey, L.A.: Chronic factitious illness: a behavioral approach. Int. Psychiat. Med. *13:* 173–184 (1983).
Lamont, J.A.: Vaginismus. Am. J. Obstet. Gynec. *131:* 632–636 (1978).
Lichtenstein, E.: The smoking problem: a behavioral perspective. J. consult. clin. Psychol. *50:* 844–819 (1982).

Lightman, S.L.; Jacobs, H.S.: Naloxone: non-steroidal treatment for postmenopausal flushing. Lancet *ii:* 1071 (1979).

Lopiccolo, J.; Lopiccolo, L.: Handbook of sex therapy (Plenum Press, New York 1978).

Lyles, J.N.; Burnish, T.G.; Krozely, M.G.; Oldham, R.K.: Efficacy of relaxation training and guided imagery in reducing the aversiveness of cancer chemotherapy. J. consult. clin. Psychol. *50:* 509–524 (1982).

McDonald, R.L.: The role of emotional factors in obstetric complications: a review. Psychosom. Med. *30:* 222–237 (1968).

Meldrum, D.R.; Shamank, I.M.; Frumar, A.M.; Tataryn, I.V.; Chang, R.J.; Judd, H.L.: Elevations in skin temperature of the finger as an objective index of postmenopausal hot flashes: a standardization of the technique. Am. J. Obstet. Gynec. *15:* 713–717 (1979).

Melzack, R.; Taenzer, P.; Feldman, P.; Kinch, R.A.: Labour is still painful after prepared childbirth training. Can. med. Ass. J. *125:* 357–363 (1981).

Molnar, G.W.: Body temperature during menopausal hot flashes. J. appl. Physiol. *38:* 499–503 (1975).

Mullen, F.C.: Treatment of a case of dysmenorrhoea by behavior therapy technique. J. nerv. ment. Dis. *147:* 371–376 (1968).

Mullen, F.C.: Treatment of dysmenorrhoea by professional and student behavior. Proc. 5th Annu. Meet. Ass. Advancement Behav. Ther., Washington, D.C., 1971.

Novaco, R.W.: Stress inoculation: a cognitive therapy for anter and its application to a case of depression. J. consult. clin. Psychol. *45:* 600–608 (1977).

Noval, E.R.; Jones, G.D.; Jones, H.W.: Gynecology (Williams & Wilkins, Baltimore 1975).

Ollendick, T.H.; Hersen, M.: Child behavioral assessment (Pergamon Press, New York 1984).

Olten, D.S.; Noonberg, A.R.: Biofeedback: clinical application in behavioral medicine (Prentice-Hall, Englewood Cliffs 1980).

Polit, D.F.; Larocco, S.A.: Social and psychological correlates of menopausal symptoms. Psychosom. Med. *42:* 335–345 (1980).

Redd, W.H.; Andresen, G.V.: Conditional aversion in cancer patients. Behav. Ther. *4:* 3–4 (1981).

Redd, W.H.; Andresen, G.V.; Minagawa, R.Y.: Hypnotic control of anticipation emesis in patients receiving cancer chemotherapy. J. consult. clin. Psychol. *50:* 14–19 (1982).

Redd, W.H.; Andrykowski, M.A.: Behavioral intervention in cancer treatment: controlling aversion reactions to chemotherapy. J. consult. clin. Psychol. *50:* 1018–1029 (1982).

Rimm, D.C.; Masters, J.C.: Behavior therapy; 2nd ed. (Academic Press, New York 1979).

Ruble, D.N.: Premenstrual symptoms: a reinterpretation. Science *197:* 191–192 (1977).

Schultz, J.H.; Luthe, W.: Autogenic training: a psychophysiological approach in psychotherapy (Grune & Stratton, New York 1959).

Stevenson, D.W.; Delprato, D.J.: Multiple component self-control program for menopausal hot flashes. J. Behav. Ther. exp. Psychiat. *14:* 137–140 (1983).

St. James-Roberts, I.; Chamberlain, G.; Haran, F.J.; Hutchinson, C.M.P.A.: Use of electromyographic and skin-conductance biofeedback relaxation training to facilitate childbirth in primiparae. J. psychosom. Res. *26:* 455–462 (1982).

St. James-Roberts, I.; Hutchinson, C.; Haran, F.J.; Chamberlain, G.: Biofeedback as an aid to childbirth. Br. J. Obstet. Gynaec. *90:* 56–60 (1983).

Tarler-Benlolo, L.: The role of relaxation in biofeedback training: a critical review of the literature. Psychol. Bull. *85:* 727–755 (1978).

Tasto, D.P.; Chesney, M.A.: Muscle relaxation treatment for primary dysmenorrhoea. Behav. Ther. 5: 668–672 (1974).

Thompson, B.; Hart, S.A.; Durno, D.: Menopausal age and symptomatology in general practice. J. biosocial Sci. 5: 71–80 (1975).

Torman, J.: Hormonal vs. psychosomatic disturbances of the menopause. Psychosomatics 9: 17–21 (1968).

Tubbs, W.; Carnahan, C.: Clinical biofeedback for primary dysmenorrhoea: a pilot study. Proc. Biofeedback Res. Soc., Colorado Springs 1976.

Turk, D.C.; Meichenbaum, D.; Genest, M.: Pain and behavioral medicine: a cognitive-behavioral perspective (Guilford Press, New York 1983).

Turner, S.M.; Calhoun, K.S.; Adams, H.E.: Handbook of clinical behavior therapy (Wiley, New York 1981).

Voda, A.M.: Climacteric hot flash. Maturitas 3: 73–90 (1981).

Walker, C.E.: Sexual disorders; in Doleys, Meredith, Ciminero, Behavioral medicine: assessment and treatment strategies (Plenum Press, New York 1982).

Whitehead, E.W.; Bosmajian, L.S.: Behavioral medicine approaches to gastrointestinal disorders. J. consult. clin. Psychol. 50: 972–983 (1982).

Winokur, G.: Depression in the menopause. Am. J. Psychiat. 130: 92–93 (1973).

Wolpe, J.: Psychotherapy by reciprocal inhibition (Stanford University Press, Stanford 1958).

Zlutnick, S.; Taylor, C.B.: Chronic pain; in Doleys, Meredith, Ciminero, Behavioral medicine: assessment and treatment strategies (Plenum Press, New York 1982).

Elizabeth A. Klonoff, PhD, Psychiatry and Neurology, Case Western Reserve University School of Medicine, Cleveland, OH 44106 (USA)

Obgynethical Issues – Present and Future

Mary B. Mahowald

Case Western Reserve University, School of Medicine, Cleveland, Ohio, USA

Two developments of the past 15 years have seldom been related, but their relationship needs to be recognized if one is to appreciate the uniqueness of obstetrics and gynecology among other medical specialties. These are (a) the progress of the women's movement or feminism, and (b) the progress of medical science and technology, particularly with regard to prenatal diagnosis and techniques for thwarting or facilitating pregnancy. By feminism I here mean the recognition that women have generally been deprived of equal opportunities with men, and the effort to rectify that situation [1]. While concurring on these points, feminists have disagreed about the best means of achieving their goal, and that disagreement has spawned conflicting ideologies within feminism [2].

As public support for the goal of sexual equality has grown, so have criticism and mistrust of medical power and technology. From a feminist perspective the criticism is especially directed towards the practice of obstetrics and gynecology, as epitomizing the inegalitarian and paternalistic nature of the physician-patient relationship [3, 4]. Recent manifestations of such criticism and response to it include the growth of the Women's Health Movement, along with books such as *Our Bodies Ourselves* [5], Arms' [6] *Immaculate Deception*, Rich's [7] *Of Woman Born*, Scully's [8] *Men Who Control Women's Health*, and Harrison's [9] *A Woman in Residence*. As with any critical movement there are excesses, inaccuracies, inconsistencies, and vagueness in its expressions, but it also provides clinicians with an important opportunity for growth in self-understanding and professional sensitivity through analysis of what is valid and invalid in these criticisms.

In this article I wish to facilitate that analysis through discussion of the factors peculiar to the specialty of obstetrics and gynecology which raise ethical questions regarding sexual equality. I also wish to survey some of the older and newer ethical issues raised by reproductive technologies, and explore several of these in greater detail. In doing so, I will discuss the main ethical principles on which the assessment of alternative positions may be based, and suggest questions which may guide their application to specific 'obgynethical' issues.

Physician-Patient Relationship

Traditionally, the physician-patient relationship, as we have already indicated, is paternalistic, i.e., it mimics the father-child relationship, in which one party is clearly powerful and autonomous, the other vulnerable and dependent [10]. Because 'father knows best' what is in the child's (patient's) best interest, he or she has not only the right, but at times the responsibility to override the wishes of the child. Moreover, the father's decisions are not simply made in behalf of an incompetent child (since some children are surely competent), or in behalf of an unconscious or extremely ill child (since most children are neither), but mainly in behalf of normal, healthy children.

Clearly, the father-knows-and-does-what-is-best image of the physician is particularly applicable to the obstetrician/gynecologist's relationship to his patient. That patient is often quite competent, conscious, and normal, yet her relationship to the physician is one of vulnerability. Because our socialization process tends to encourage men to be dominant and women to accept that dominance, the fact that the physician is usually male while the patient is always female serves to reinforce the inegalitarian nature of the relationship [11].

Further compromising the situation of the woman-as-patient is the fact that matters to be discussed with an obstetrician/gynecologist are often quite intimate (life-style, sexual practices and relationships), and no similar personal revelations are required or expected on the part of the physician. Such topics are typically more integral to the patient's self-concept than are conditions treated by other specialties. Not infrequently, they raise important moral questions for both patient and clinician. Moreover, where the patient is pregnant, her situation is significantly complicated by the fact that her physician may view his primary responsibility as extended to 2 individuals whose interests and needs may be incompatible.

Precisely because a traditional interpretation of the obstetrician's role is that he has 2 patients from the beginning (if not before) to the end of the pregnancy, ethical decisions in this specialty are inseparable from legal and social questions. For example, the *Roe v. Wade* decision of the US Supreme Court in 1973 challenges the traditional 2-patient concept of obstetrics, by affirming the legal right of a woman to terminate a pregnancy during the first two trimesters [12]. Thus, the role concept of the professional may be at odds with the legal system. Further, since the state is said to have an interest in the fetus which commences at viability, the technology which has advanced viability into the second trimester may occasion a change in existing law, such that state interest in the fetus may override the choice of the pregnant woman at what ever point viability occurs.

Decisions regarding fertility and infertility constitute a major portion of the ethical decisions made by patients and clinicians in an obstetrics/ gynecology practice. Clearly, such decisions impact on women's lives more than on men's, even if we allow that fathers are equally responsible for their children. It is inevitably and exclusively women's bodies that are affected by pregnancy, childbirth and lactation; it is not inevitable but it is empirically true that most women bear most of the responsibility for raising children [7, 13].

Since the participation of men in the process of childbirth is a comparatively recent phenomenon, it is not surprising that some women resist the medicalization of the event, as signifying masculine control of an essentially female capability [7]. Indeed, some have read the motivation of men choosing obstetrics/gynecology as their specialty as a way of reducing the lack of power they experience in confronting the origin of life [14]. No man can 'make' a baby, but men have made women bear children, even against their will. Recent court decisions requiring women to undergo cesarean section delivery for apparent fetal distress illustrate that power on a social level [15]. Resistance to the revival of midwifery practices supports the suspicion that men wish to maintain the level of control achieved in obstetrical practice [6, 16].

In general, feminists decry a double standard regarding the social responsibilities and expectations of women and men. Those who work outside the home return to domestic responsibilities in which some men assist, but few share equally [17]. That women's work, whether in or outside the home, is prevalently viewed as less important than the work of men is reflected in salary discrepancies between the sexes, and in the low pay and regard given for child care and housework [18, 19]. This attitude may be expressed in the physician-patient relationship through disregard for women's time: the assumption that women-patients must wait because the physician's time is more valuable. Another frequent assumption is that women are more concerned about their appearance than are men. Where this is true, whether the trait is natural or nurtured, it may negatively affect a woman's self-concept during the course of a pregnancy, and exacerbate the psychological toll of surgical interventions such as breast removal for metastatic cancer. A double standard is also evident in the use of first names for patients, who address their physicians by title and last name. Admittedly, such a double standard is often reinforced from both sides of the relationship.

It may be argued that the physician-patient relationship is essentially inegalitarian, and that the practice of obstetrics/gynecology merely instances that relationship without any ethical implications, sexist or otherwise. In other words, the fact that more obstetrician/gynecologists are male and their patients female does not imply sexism; and inequality, if based on fact, does not constitute a moral problem. The soundness of this argument hinges on the concept of equality which it assumes [20]. If equality is construed as sameness (and inequality, correspondingly, as difference), then obviously the physician-patient relationship, or obstetrician/gynecologist's relationship to a patient, or for that matter any person's relationship to any other person, is inegalitarian – because all of us are different. Surely the differences in themselves are morally neutral: it is the values assigned to them that move us into an ethical context, where moral conflicts may arise. Equality thus represents either the same or different traits or accomplishments as having the same values; inequality means that they do not. The justification of equality or inequality as a moral state of affairs depends ultimately on some principle of justice, by which each person is valued as a person, and the differing abilities, needs, and autonomy of individuals are respected in a plan of distribution of limited resources.

On such an account of equality or justice, inequality in the physician-patient relationship only presents a moral problem if relevant differences between the two are *not* respected, or either party is not valued by the other as a person. Where sexism occurs, it means that sexuality is used irrelevantly as a criterion for distinguishing between people. Indeed, in this age of antimedical backlash, reverse sexism is also a distinct possibility [21]. Accordingly, an ideal of justice which respects differences while distributing resources fairly provides a useful vantage point from which to reassess the physician-patient relationship as well as ethical issues in the practice of obstetrics and gynecology.

Persistent Ethical Issues

'Obgynethical' issues run the gamut of ethical issues raised in other medical specialties, e. g., questions of truth-telling, confidentiality, consent to experimental therapy, criteria for determination of death, allocation of scarce medical resources. But those peculiar to obstetrics/gynecology have mainly to do with reproduction, either curbing or enhancing it. Recurrent themes include the right and responsibility to reproduce or not to reproduce, the right and responsibility to assist others to reproduce or not to reproduce, and rights and responsibilities concerning sexual expression and gender identity. Complicating some of these themes is the range of age and competence in which such issues may be addressed by patients and their families. The fact that the physiological capability for reproduction is present in children as well as in retarded mentally ill adults expands our responsibility of care for them to their potential offspring. Motherhood constitutes legal emancipation for some minors, but clearly does not establish that the new mother is adequate to assume the responsibility of primary care-giver for her newborn [22].

Ethical questions concerning curtailment of pregnancy, especially abortion, have been dealt with rather extensively in philosophical literature. With regard to sterilization and contraception the concerns invoked are often based on the principle of informed consent, the right to express one's sexuality without the risk of pregnancy, and responsibility to the larger society, including other family members and future generations [23]. 'Natural law' arguments, i. e., those which assume that reproduction is a natural process that ought not to be interfered with, are also offered [24]. Similar claims are made with regard to abortion. Here, however, the moral status of the fetus is usually perceived as crucial to ethical assessment, and the right of the pregnant woman to control what transpires within her own body is also stressed [25, 26].

From a clinical perspective, an individual may wish to separate his or her own moral stance from that of the patient, allowing the latter to choose a course at variance with one's own. This implies some tolerance for what the clinician perceives as wrong, or else ambivalence regarding what he or she believes is right. Unless we posit a dichotomy between professional and moral responsibility (by which the physician sheds one skin for another in commuting between hospital and home), there surely is need to reconcile the two. In other words, we need to determine how to act both morally and professionally with patients with whom we have ethical disagreements regarding clinical decisions. Typically, such disagreements reflect moderate rather than extreme positions on the part of physicians – for example, one who considers early abortion morally justified if a pregnancy is unwanted, who nonetheless considers it wrong to choose or to perform a second trimester abortion because the fetus is not of the desired sex. There is an admirable consistency in the position of the ardent pro-life physician who not only refuses to perform abortions but organizes lobbying efforts to eliminate liberal abortion statutes; there is a similarly admirable consistency on the part of the pro-choice clinician who operates a free abortion clinic, and lobbies against restrictive abortion laws. But consistency is surely not a sufficient basis for honoring the practices of either individual. Beyond consistency, each of us needs to confront and evaluate the reasons which support our practice.

Some of the ire that debate about abortion evokes might be assuaged through broader recognition of the extreme complexity of certain cases. Often the image of abortion in the mind of the militant antiabortionist is a late stage decision for a trivial reason; and the image in the mind of the militant proabortionist is a procedure judged necessary for the life or well-being of the pregnant woman [27]. Many of those who concur with antiabortionists regarding the former situation, agree with proabortionists in the latter case. It is the situations that lie between these positions that are most problematic, since that is where those who cherish *both* life and liberty more often confront the dilemma of having to choose between the two. The value of (fetal) life is then more apt to conflict with the value of autonomy as applicable to the patient and/or to clinicians.

Legally, there are limits to what patients and clinicians may do, but these do not resolve the moral dilemmas of individuals. Even for those who consider the abortion issue settled, other ethical questions are inevitable. For example, how should a physician respond to the queries of the mother of a sexually active teenager, also his patient, concerning the daughter's possible practice of contraception? Or how should a clinician deal with a patient's request to sterilize his moderately retarded child? In such situations, there are no predefined, fixed, or exclusive ways of acting morally; yet this does not imply that whatever one does is morally justified. In ethics, as in clinical practice, we assume that the application of reason to the nuances of the situation, especially when conjoined to the rational input of others, will bring us closer to the correct solution. Just as patient diagnosis entails consideration of different bodily systems, so 'ethical diagnosis' entails analysis of basic ethical principles. And just as therapeutic prescriptions are never certain to be successful, although that is surely their intent, so ethical decisions are never certain to be correct answers to the questions asked, although that is their intent.

Applicable Principles

What are the ethical principles or 'systems' to be checked out in determining ethical 'prescriptions'? Basically, there are four: the principles of beneficence, autonomy, truthfulness, and justice [28]. As abstract as these may sound, each represents a certain content that clinicians and patients alike may apply to ethical quandaries. Like bodily systems, they overlap, but our understanding of the whole is enhanced through their separate consideration.

The first, beneficence, is essentially embodied in the Hippocratic imperative: 'to help, or at least to do no harm' [29]. Accordingly, this principle comprises both positive and negative duties towards the patient. The latter are sometimes described under the rubric of nonmaleficence, which represents a more stringent obligation than simple beneficence. Practically, however, it may not only be difficult but unhelpful to observe this distinction, because the very 'doing of harm' constitutes the 'doing of good' to particular patients. Insofar as medical and surgical interventions are therapeutic, they are all of this type. However, it remains the task of individuals to determine the proportion of harms and benefits which is expected, so that the minimal criterion of an equal balance between the two is observed. Beyond that point of obligation, virtue invites the practitioner to do 'more good', that is, to do more than what is minimally required legally or morally in behalf of the patient as well as others [30]. In applying this principle to specific cases, therefore, the practitioner asks: 'Is my intervention justified on the basis of the good result expected primarily for the patient(s), and secondarily for others affected?' The answer to this question provides an important consequentialist or utilitarian input into the decision-making process.

The next two principles, autonomy and truthfulness, are essentially 'deontological', that is, a priori, or based on nonconsequentialist rules or laws that arise from the very meaning of human nature or from divine command. Such principles are held to be discernible by human beings through their use of reason or faith (or both), and universally applicable and binding. In our own day, the principle of autonomy embodied in the concept of 'informed consent' has widely replaced the traditional paternalistic model of the physician's role. Important as it is, this concept applies the principle of autonomy to only one of those influenced by clinical ethical decisions, namely, the competent patient. In obstetrical and other reproductive decisions, however, there is often another autonomous individual affected, namely the putative or possible father. Moreover, clinicians themselves surely do not surrender their own autonomy at the door of the treatment or operating room. They are responsible for what they do and do not do, regardless of what the patient chooses. To base decisions exclusively on the patient's 'informed consent' is to ignore that ongoing responsibility, and subscribe to a purely instrumentalist interpretation of the physician's role. To base decisions on the broader principle of autonomy is to ask the question: 'What course does each of the individuals who will be affected by this decision prefer?' Where there are conflicting answers, these need to be weighed according to the degree in which the individuals will be affected. Among patients themselves, who are surely more significantly affected than others, that significance is not always of equal weight.

Since autonomous decisions can only be made on the basis of correct understanding of alternatives and their implications, the principle of truthfulness, or an ideal of truth-telling, is closely related to autonomy. There is a sense, of course, in which truth-telling is an impossible goal, because of the inevitable limitations of knowledge and ability to communicate. What remains possible is truthfulness, as an effort to understand and communicate to others accurately. As with autonomy, the obligation to be truthful extends to all of those who have truth to tell, and not only to physicians vis-à-vis their patients. It does not imply, however, that any individual has a right to any truth that another holds. A clearly justified limitation to truth-telling is recognition of the right to privacy of the individual about whom the truth is known. In other words, there is also an obligation to observe confidentiality, which is especially applicable to the kinds of information that an obstetrician-gynecologist possesses. The pertinent question for the clinician, therefore, is two-faceted: 'What information do I owe my patient, those close to her, and other health professionals, and what information am I obligated not to disclose?'

Another practical question immediately follows: 'How might I most effectively communicate or refrain from communicating, where circumstances call for either approach?'

The fourth ethical 'system' to be checked out in determining responses to ethical dilemmas is the principle of justice. This may be construed as deontological or utilitarian, and as applicable either to individual decisions or social policy. In either case, it is the notion of distributive (rather than retributive) justice about which we are concerned. Macroallocation decisions regarding distribution of health care resources are mainly a matter of social policy, but microallocation decisions are made every day through determinations regarding time, space, equipment, expertise, and medication.

If the principle of justice is to be applied in obstetrics, some determination needs to be made regarding the status of the fetus, so that conflicts that pit the alleged rights of the fetus against those of the pregnant woman may be addressed in that light. Where fetus and pregnant woman count equally as patients or persons, justice requires that neither has the greater claim against the other, and a random way of determining care for one as opposed to the other may be acceptable [31]. Even then, however, duties towards, and effects on others are morally relevant when the rights of persons are in conflict. On the other hand, justice does not require equal consideration of fetus and pregnant woman if either of the following positions is maintained: (a) 'rights' to life and liberty are proportionate to the developmental status of the individual, whether that individual counts as person or not; and (b) the 'personhood' by which an individual is judged worthy of equitable treatment with other persons commences at birth or some later point of life.

Since 1973 the US Supreme Court has upheld a view not quite like either of the above. According to that ruling, the state has a legitimate interest in the welfare of the fetus commencing at viability, which usually occurs during the third trimester. Prior to that point in fetal development, safe abortions are permissible on the basis of a woman's choice. Subsequently, her choice may be subordinated to the fetus' right to survive. The concept of justice invoked here is one which entails equal treatment for all who are legally persons, and a construal or viability as constituting legal personhood. Only when the life or health of the pregnant woman is threatened may a viable fetus' life be terminated through abortion. In other words, life and liberty are not viewed as equal values of those who count as persons before the law; justice implies that life is the more basic

basic right or value, whose denial may not be permitted in the name of another's liberty.

Newer Ethical Issues

Recently, the courts have ordered cesarean sections to be performed on women who had declined consent for the surgery. The grounds for these rulings were the indication of fetal distress through prenatal monitoring [15]. Clearly such cases represent even greater restrictions to women's autonomy than do statutes prohibiting third trimester abortions. Again, an interpretation of justice as entailing equal treatment of all persons, and as extended to viable fetuses as 'legal persons', may be invoked to justify the violence and risk which major surgery represents. Positions which affirm the rights of the pregnant woman over those of the fetus may also be maintained under the aegis of justice, and these seem more defensible in a society which prevalently upholds the rights of individuals to control their own lives and bodies.

Several additional factors argue against these legal decisions. First, the risk undergone in major surgery is real, even though less than that which some fetuses may undergo through vaginal delivery. Second, the Roe v. Wade decision of 1973 asserts that the state does *not* have a compelling interest in preserving the life of viable fetuses if 'the life or health of the mother' is endangered by carrying the child to term [12]. And third, no parent has ever been required by law to undergo surgery or general anesthesia (e. g., bone marrow or kidney transplant) to save the life of his dying child, who is surely a person. Obviously, court orders for coercive cesarean sections apply their interpretation of justice to women only. It may well be that justice demands not a repudiation of the position itself (that viable fetuses should be protected even if this entails risk to the pregnant woman), but simply its extension to the other half of the human community, and to all those who are indispensable to support of other human lives. In deciding among conflicting interests, therefore, the pertinent question for clinicians and patients alike is the following: 'Which approach is most likely to effect an equitable distribution of harms and benefits among those concerned?'

Recent developments in fertility research have evoked recognition of ethical questions surrounding marital and sexual relationships, parenthood, and the right to biologically related progeny. Some of these issues have been with us for a long time, without raising much public concern – perhaps because the controversial practices (such as artificial insemination by husband or donor) are usually implemented covertly. Newer means of facilitating reproduction tend to focus on infertility in women rather than men, and in that context, successful interventions can hardly be covert – e. g., when a woman who has long been infertile is suddenly pregnant, or when a nonpregnant woman brings home the newborn of her husband and a 'surrogate'. In time, as techniques are refined and routinized, confidentiality may be better maintained in cases of ovum transfer and in vitro fertilization, as in artificial insemination. However, in all of these situations, a rather new metaethical question is raised, namely, 'Whose child is this?'

The question is important ethically because its answer specifies a relationship which connotes rights and responsibilities. In a certain sense, all who assist in the development, birth, and nurturance of a child are 'parents'. That is, they have helped that person to *become* and to *be* in the world. Without Drs. *Steptoe* and *Edwards,* for example, *Louise Brown* would never have existed; so their role is not entirely unlike that of biological parents [32]. The donors of ovum and sperm are obviously the genetic parents of the developing fetus and future child. Although there is no direct contact between them and the fertilized ovum, their empirical contribution remains crucial and influential. In contrast to sperm donation, ovum transfer requires medical intervention and entails some risk and discomfort. These factors are clearly more significant in the relationship between the surrogate who is also the ovum donor and the developing fetus – because of the prolonged period of fetal dependence, with accompanying conspicuousness and physical costs. In all of these cases, if there were not social or moral inhibition against sexual intercourse between donor and host-parent, that procedure might be preferred to artificial insemination, as indeed both safer and more 'natural'.

From an ethical standpoint, just as we may stress the nurturant role of adoptive parents, we need to take account – as a matter of justice and truthfulness – of the significant role played by others in the birth of some infants. To the extent that their contribution is demanding of them and crucial to the infant, they are to that degree 'parents'. Thus, the adoptive, genetically unrelated parent who cares for a child through the first 18 years of life is more parent to that child than the medical student who donates sperm for artificial insemination of an unknown woman. But the 'surrogate' mother who contributes ovum and uterus for a period of 9 months is also more of a parent than the medical student.

Accordingly, the adoptive parent in the former case, and the surrogate in the latter case, maintain a certain right to influence decisions regarding the fate of the child or fetus. Adoptive parents may arguably overrule a biological parent's decision with regard to their child, where they have nurtured the child for most of his or her life. Surrogate mothers may decide during a pregnancy to have an abortion, or to keep their biologically related infants as their own [33, 34]. Legal conflicts are possible in both situations (e. g., suit for breach of contract, or for transference of custody), but the ethical question on which their resolution appropriately depends remains the same: 'Whose child (fetus) is this?' As we anticipate yet more complicated arrangements through technological advances, this question achieves even greater significance. Consider, for example, the possibility of a surrogate mother, whose pregnancy was initiated through the implantation of a blastocyst formed through in vitro fertilization of donor ovum and sperm, delivering an infant to be given to an infertile couple as their adopted child. We might extend the complexity of the case even further by positing a lesbian couple, or a single man or woman as the adoptive parents. Whether marriage, and/or a loving relationship, is essential to moral assessment of the situation is problematic. None of these possibilities is empirically unavailable, and all of them have been defended on moral grounds.

In an individualistic society such as ours, the concept of parenthood is often quite traditional and biological: a heterosexual married couple who conceive a child through sexual intercourse, each contributing 23 chromosomes, one contributing her uterus, along with the physical and emotional costs of pregnancy and childbirth, both partners contributing thereafter to the child's nurturance. In some way, the child is then looked upon as the property of the parents: he or she *belongs* to them, is named by them, is kept and cared for by them unless 'given up' for adoption, or until (in the case of daughters) 'given away' in marriage to be kept and cared for by another. Admittedly, parental rights over children have legal as well as moral limits, but they remain extremely significant determinants of children's lives and identities. Moreover, through the nuclear families which our modern transient life-style has entailed, the family unit has come to represent an end itself, a kind of self-justifying system. Within that framework it is difficult to appreciate a more complicated and extended concept of parenthood.

To grapple adequately with the ethical questions which advances in reproductive technologies present, we need to examine our traditional concept of parenthood in light of the fact that in many cases it takes more than 2 individuals to develop a child. That fact already points to rights and responsibilities on the part of the developers, and to conflicts in the exercise of those rights and responsibilities. The principle of justice suggests that such conflicts might be resolved through examination of the differing contributions of parent figures, including the duration, depth, and demands of their relationship to the child. A 'priority among parents' might be determined on the basis of their nurturant input, whether physical, psychological, or both.

Another ethical principle that is relevant here is beneficence, i. e., the benefits owed to nonautonomous as well as autonomous persons. Surely, the parent-child relationship occurs between persons rather than between a person and an object. That status clearly limits the control that may legally or morally be exercised by parents over their children [35]. Beneficence describes the limit as an obligation to do good and avoid harm to another. There is thus no absolute right to *have* a child; whatever right there is to parenthood is morally limited by the extent to which the parental relationship will be beneficent or at least not maleficent towards the child. The same may be said for the right or responsibility to assist another in having a child.

Justice is in a certain sense an extension of the principle of beneficence: an equitable distribution of harms and benefits. Applying this to reproductive technologies entails examination of the costs of developing and implementing the technologies, and their accessibility to the general population. As long as certain ways of facilitating reproduction are available only to a limited number of those in need (those who can pay for them), it may hardly be claimed that biological reproduction is a recognized, universal right. Limited application of technology may be justified on the basis of its experimental status, but justice demands that the discrepancies in accessibility be reduced as much as possible. That the well-off receive the benefits of the research may be defended on utilitarian grounds: since someone has to pay the cost, current discrimination practice is necessary as a means of accomplishing its universal availability. It would seem, however, that the ideal of justice might be approximated even now. Since the technology is of such great benefit to a wealthy few, part of what those few pay might be directed to the purchase of its availability to some of the poor. Although this view may be incompatible with the self-interested motivation of a free-enterprise system, it is not inconsistent with the democratic demands of justice. Similar arguments have been made regarding the availability of abortion and contraceptive procedures.

Conclusion

At the outset I suggested that analysis of current feminist criticism of the medical profession in general, and of obstetrics/gynecology in particular, might yield helpful insights for clinical practice. The same may be said for the women's movement. In fact, I believe the question 'Whose children are they?' is crucial to understanding and assessment of different versions of feminism – as well as antifeminism [36]. Advances in reproductive technologies have not only increased the capacity of individuals to control their reproductive lives, they have greatly complicated the expression of that capacity. Individualistic versions of feminism and medicine (i.e., those which focus on individual women or patients) have accented the former, while 'communalistic' versions (i.e., those which are concerned with the larger community) accent the latter [37]. 'Whose child?' is answered individualistically as 'Mine'. From a communalistic perspective, the answer is 'Ours'. The first response implies that the answerer has full rights and total responsibility for the child; the second implies shared rights and responsibilities. Increasingly, the first answer is unrealizable, and the second is empirically unavoidable but morally problematic.

As medicine has moved towards a more socialized understanding of itself, and individual physicians have observed their responsibility to patients as extending to the broader society, American feminism has reflected a critique of individualism, even while emphasizing the reproductive rights of the individual [21, 38]. Conflicting ideologies, whether in medicine or feminism, are not likely to be resolved any sooner than the perennial metaphysical problem of 'the one and the many' [39]; but some of the tension between them may be reduced and rendered constructive through recognition of the validity and inadequacy of mutually exclusive positions. To the question 'Whose child is this?' the answers 'Mine' and 'Ours' are both valid and inadequate. 'Mine' is surely least inadequately applied to the biological mother who has nurtured her child beyond pregnancy to some stage of self-sufficiency; but even here, the man through whom the child was conceived and who shared in the child's nurturance may also call the child 'Mine'. Thus the couple together, less inadequately, say 'Our'. To the extent that others share the joy and burden of nurturing children, they too, even less inadequately, join in the 'Our'.

My own view, therefore, of the best justified version of feminism is coincident with what I believe to be the best justified view of the physician-patient relationship. It is egalitarian in that it entails recognition of the personhood status of women and men, physicians and patients alike. It is pragmatic in that it attempts to mediate between individualistic and communalistic emphases, between empiricist and rationalist concerns, and between practical and idealistic elements of conflicting views [40]. The mediation entails a critical, ongoing effort to apply basic ethical principles to concrete situations. Beneficence, autonomy, truthfulness, and justice are the principles; persons or potential persons describe the concrete situation as a complex of interactions. Just as prescriptions based on diagnosis and prognosis are never absolutely certain to provide correct solutions, this is also true with regard to moral dilemmas in medicine. But our faith in human reason, the principles we apply, and in the efficacy of collaborative effort to bring us closer to the truth may be verified here also – as advances in reproductive biology continue to raise ethical questions.

References

1 Jaggar, A.: On sexual equality. Ethics *84:*275–292 (1974).
2 Jaggar, A.: Political philosophies of women's liberation; in Bishop, Weinzweig, Philosophy and women, pp. 258–265 (Wadsworth, Belmont 1979).
3 Holmes, H.B.: The birth of a women-centered analysis; in Holmes, Hoskins, Gross, Birth control and controlling birth, pp. 5–6 (Humana, Clifton 1979).
4 Peterson, S.R.: The politics of prenatal diagnosis; in Holmes, Hoskins, Gross, Birth control and controlling birth, pp. 98–104 (Humana, Clifton 1979).
5 Boston Women's Health Course Collective: Our bodies ourselves (New England Free Press, Boston 1971).
6 Arms, S.: Immaculate deception (Bantam, New York 1975).
7 Rich, A.: Of woman born (Bantam, New York 1977).
8 Scully, D.: Men who control women's health (Houghton-Mifflin, Boston 1980).
9 Harrison, M.: A women in residence (Random House, New York 1982).
10 Childress, J.: What is paternalism?; in Robison, Pritchard, Medical responsibilities, pp. 18–21 (Humana, Clifton 1979).
11 Bidese, C.M.; Danais, D.G.: Physician characteristics and distribution in the U.S.; 1981 ed., pp. 14, 15 (American Medical Association, Chicago 1982).
12 Roe v. Wade majority opinion, United States Supreme Court, January 22, 1973. 410 U.S. 113, 93 S. Ct. 705.
13 Breslau, N.: Care of disabled children and women's time use. Med. Care *21:* 620–629 (1983).
14 Ehrenreich, B.; English, D.: Witches, midwives and nurses: a history of women healers, pp. 12–15 (Feminist Press, Old Westbury 1973).
15 Annas, G.: Forced cesareans: the most unkindest cut. Hastings Center Rep. *12:* 16–17, 45 (1982).
16 Leeson, J.; Gray, J.: Women and medicine, pp. 52–56 (Tavistock, London 1978).

17 Scott, H.: Does socialism liberate women?, pp. 199–200 (Beacon, Boston 1974).
18 Illich, I.: Gender, pp. 24, 174 (Pantheon, New York 1982).
19 Ratner, R.S..: Equal employment policy for women: strategies for implementation in the USA, Canada and Western Europe, pp. 20–23 (Temple, Philadelphia 1978).
20 Blackstone, W. (ed.): The concept of equality (Burgess, Minneapolis 1969).
21 Starr, P.: The social transformation of American medicine, pp. 379–419 (Basic Books, New York 1982).
22 Leikin, S.: Minors' assent or dissent to medical treatment. J. Pediat. 102: 169–176 (1983).
23 Petchesky, R.: Reproductive freedom: beyond 'a woman's right to choose'. Signs: J. Women Culture Society 5: 661–685 (1980).
24 Curran, C.E.: Natural law and contemporary moral theology (chapter 2), and Sexuality and sin (chapter 3), pp. 97–158, 159–188; in Curran, Contemporary problems in moral theology (Fides, Notre Dame 1970).
25 Sumner, L.W.: Abortion and moral theory, pp. 26–33, 40–123 (Princeton 1981).
26 Nicholson, S.: Abortion and the Roman Catholic Church, pp. 1–39 (Religious Ethics, Knoxville 1978).
27 Mahowald, M.B.: Towards continuing the dialogue. Cross Currents 29: 330–335 (1979).
28 Beauchamp, T.; Childress, J.: Principles of biomedical ethics (Oxford, New York 1979).
29 Selections from the Hippocratic corpus; in Reiser, Dyck, Curran, Ethics in medicine, p. 7 (MIT, Cambridge 1977).
30 Callahan, D.: Minimalist ethics. Hastings Center Rep. 11: 19–25 (1981).
31 Childress, J.: Who shall live when not all shall live?, in Muson, Intervention and reflection, pp. 501–504 (Wadsworth, Belmont 1983).
32 Keiffer, G.H.: Reproductive technology: the state of the art; in Mappes, Zembaty, Biomedical ethics, p. 487.
33 Riccardi, M.; Webb, G.: Ohio surrogate: 'It all happened so fast.' Plain Dealer, Cleveland, pp. 1, 2-B (Nov. 3, 1983).
34 Krimmel, H.T.: The case against surrogate parenting. Hastings Center Rep. 13: 35–39 (1983).
35 Robertson, J.: Legal aspects of withholding medical treatment from handicapped children; in Doudera, Peters, Legal and ethical aspects of treating critically ill and terminally ill patients, pp. 214–217 (AUPHA, Ann Arbor 1982).
36 Jaggar, A.; Struhl, P.: Feminist frameworks, pp. 206–259 (McGraw-Hill, New York 1978).
37 Mahowald, M.B.: Feminism: individualistic or communalistic? Proc. Am. Cath. Phil. Ass., pp. 219–229 (1976).
38 Gilligan, C.: In a different voice (Harvard, Cambridge 1982).
39 James, W.: The one and the many; in Pragmatism, pp. 89–108 (Meridian, Cleveland 1955).
40 Mahowald, M.B.: An idealistic pragmatism, p. 176 (Nijhoff, The Hague 1972).

Mary B. Mahowald, PhD, Case Western Reserve University School of Medicine, Cleveland, OH 44106 (USA)

Subject Index

Abortion
  ethical issues 170, 171
  status of fetus 174
Acetylcholine 16
ACTH, stress 31
Adolescent mothers
  breast-feeding
    attitudes 88, 89
    incidence 84
    support systems 85
  pregnancy
    performance 81, 82
    perinatal mortality 82
    physical readiness 82
    social concerns 85–87
Adoptive parent, ethics and legal issues 176, 177
Adrenalectomy 36
Aldosterone 47
Amenorrhea
  'critical weight' hypothesis 25, 26
  hyperprolactinemia 31
  hypothalamic mechanism 30
  low weight 30
  psychogenic 29
Amniocentesis 94, 99
Ampullary-isthmic junction 13
Androgen
  intrauterine contamination 65
  menopause, levels/source 37
  receptors 8
  synthesis, theca cells 14
Androgenital syndrome 65
Androstenedione
  estrone, peripheral aromatization 37
  postmenopause, source 37
Anger, premenstrual 155, 156
Angiotensin I 47
Anovulation hyperprolactinemia 31
Anxiety-depression syndrome 43, 44
Arcuate nucleus
  dopamine-secreting neurons 20
  GnRH secretion 17
Aromatase enzyme 11
Arteriosclerotic heart disease 41
Artificial insemination
  donor semen (AID)
    children, effects 119
    contractual agreements 114
    donor requirements 115
    emotional aspects 117–119
    indications for consideration 114
    insemination procedure 115, 116
    legal problems
      adultery? 108
      child's legal status 108, 109
      physician's liability 109
    success rate, factors 116
  husband semen (AIH)
    indications for consideration 111–113
    psychiatric evaluation 113
    success rate, factors 112–114

Subject Index

Artificial insemination (cont.)
  process
    indications 110, 111
    social and psychological implications 110
    sperm collection/storage 110, 112
  religious opinion 107, 108
  technique and terminology 105, 106
Atresia 8, 9, 36

Behavior therapy
  biofeedback 153, 161
  cognitive techniques 154
  operant conditioning 151
  systematic desensitization 152
Beneficence, reproductive technologies 178
Bioethics 3
Biogenic amines
  brain neurotransmitters 28
    situation/emotional distress 30
  phenethylamine (PEA) 30
Bleeding abnormalities 5
Body temperature, hot flashes 40
Breast cancer, estrogens, role 46
Breast-feeding
  emotional aspects 2
  infant feeding, advances 83, 84
  mother's age 81
    adolescent 82

Cancer chemotherapy, anticipatory nausea/emesis 161
Cardiovascular disease 42, 48
Catecholamines 5, 21
Cesarean section, court-ordered 175
Childbearing
  delayed 2
  infertility 93, 94, 100
  optimal age 93
  psychological problems, preconception concerns 92
  term pregnancy/abortion
    amniocentesis 94, 99
    ultrasound examination 94, 95, 99
Chorionic gonadotropin, luteal function, influence 15

Clitoris
  inferior penis?, Freud 60
  orgasm 138
Communication 61
Contraception
  ethical issues 170
  guilt and disappointment 102
Corpus luteum
  function failure 12
  life span 14
  luteinized granulosa cell 14
  regression 15
Couvade syndrome 141
Cumulus cells 13

Depression, premenstrual, treatment 155
Dopamine
  FSH, LH, prolactin, effect 20
  GnRH inhibition 20, 29
  hypothalamic neurotransmitter 16
  midcycle LH surge, suppression 30
Dysmenorrhea
  behavior relaxation therapy 154, 155
  vasopressin, stress-associated 31
Dyspareunia, systematic desensitization 157

Endomentrium
  carcinoma
    long-term exogenous estrogen 45
    prevention 45
  hyperplasia, estrogen-related 45
  menstrual cycle 5
Endoplasmic reticulum 17
Endorphins 21
  LH suppression 30
  release, stress response 31
Estradiol
  bioavailability 37
  postmenopausal levels 31
  secretion, corpus luteum 14
Estrogen
  corpus luteum regression 15
  endometrial hyperplasia/carcinoma 45
  follicle regression 5, 6
  FSH synergism, action 12
  GnRH inhibition 17, 18
    pituitary sensitivity 15

Estrogen (cont.)
  granulosa cell growth 10, 11
  lipoproteins, effect 47
  long-term replacement
    contraindications 47
    indications 48
    management 48, 49
      cyclical 48
      sequential progesterone 48
  menopause 40–42
    complications 45–50
  oophorectomy, levels 36
  osteoporosis 40, 41, 48
  ovarian failure 48
  production 21
  progesterone antagonism 14
  receptors, granulosa cells 8, 12
  sexual drive, relationship 137
  thrombophlebitis 47
Estrogen-progestagen, endometrial cancer,
  protective action 45

Female sexuality
  core gender identity 60–64
  Freud's concept 58, 59
  new approaches 60
  tomboy behavior 65
Femininity
  phallic period 64
  primary stage 62
Feminism, conflicts 166–168
Fertility, ethical decisions 168
α-Fetoprotein 94
Fetus
  sex determination 95, 100
  viable, term, 'legal person' 175
Follicle-stimulating hormone (FSH)
  dopamine, effect 20
  FSH-estrogen synergism 12
  GnRH, effects 17, 18
  midcycle surge 12
  ovulation cycle 6
  postmenopause 38
  receptors, granulosa cell 8

Gallbladder disease
  estrogen replacement 47
  oral contraception 47
Gap junction 8
Gender identity
  androgen, excessive, effects 65
  chromosome abnormalities, role 66
  developmental processes 63
  disorders 68
  environmental hypothesis 62, 66, 67
  organic brain defects 66
  prenatal hormones 64, 65
  self-representation 63, 64
  tomboy 65
Golgi apparatus 17
Gonadotropin
  cyclicity, prolactin suppression 31
  follicle development, role 21
  pituitary synthesis/release 17, 22
  postmenopausal 38
  secretion, GnRH effects 19
Gonadotropin-releasing hormone (GnRH)
  activity 16, 17
  concentrations 19
  control mechanisms 19
  deficiency, naloxone effect 31
  follicle growth/ovulation 20
  ovalation cycle 6, 15
  preovulatory LH surge, influence 15, 18
  pulsed
    frequency 18
    ovulation cycle control 20
  release 29
  secretory neurons 17
  synthesis and transport 17, 18
    control mechanisms 21
Graafian follicle see Ovary
Granulosa cells
  aromatase enzyme 11
  cumulus cells 13
  estrogen
    effects 10, 11
    receptors 11
  follicle growth, third stage 10
  FSH receptors 8, 11
  luteinization 14

Hermaphroditism 67, 68
High-risk obstetrics 71

Subject Index

Histamine 16
Homosexuality 61, 65
Hot flashes
  behavioral manifestations 39
  hypothalamic-pituitary-ovarian axis 39
  incidence, symptoms, mechanism 38
  physiological components 39
  self-perception/emotional factors 160
  treatment
    behavioral approaches, stress/temperature control 159, 160
    estrogen/nonhormonal medications 159
    estrogen replacement
      alternative medications 50
      contraindications 47
      management 48
      route of administration 49
H-Y antigen factor 67
Hyperprolactinemia 31
Hypertension 46
Hypothalamic-pituitary-ovarian axis 19
Hypothalamus
  blood flow from pituitary 16
  dopaminergic activity
    deficiency 32
    hyperfunction 30
  GnRH
    pituitary response 15
    regulation 29
    secreting neurons 17
    secretion, factors modifying 22
  hormones, action
    modification factors 5
    pituitary 5
Hysterectomy, psychological effects 141, 143

Infertility
  ethical decisions 168
  psychological implications 102, 103, 113
  sexual dysfunction 114
  sperm, antibodies/autoantibodies 113
    artificial insemination 113
  stress 29, 111–114

Limbic system
  activity 28
  'emotional brain' 29
Lipids
  hepatic metabolism 47
  lipoproteins: HDL, LDL, VLDL 47
Luteinizing hormone (LH)
  dopamine, effect 20
  GnRH 16, 17
  ovulation cycle 6, 12, 13, 30
  pituitary release
    pulsatile 18
    relationship to hot flashes 39
  postmenopause 38
  serum levels, naloxone 31
  surge, GnRH effect 17, 18
  theca cell 11
Luteinizing hormone-releasing hormone (LH-RH) 4

Mastectomy, sexuality modifications 144, 145
Melanocyte-stimulating hormone (MSH) 31, 32
Menarche 26
Menopause
  defeminization 38
  endocrinological changes
    androgens 37
    estrogens 37, 40, 42
  osteoporosis 40
  physiological changes 38
  psychological problems 43, 44
  skin changes 42, 43
  treatment
    estrogen replacement 40, 42
      complications 45
      reassurance 44
  vaginal atrophy 42
Menses
  alterations, exercise-associated 25, 26
  factors shaping adolescent's view 25
Menstrual cycle
  disorders, psychosomatic considerations 2
  dysfunction
    exercise-associated 5, 26

Menstrual cycle (cont.)
  dysfunction
    psychosomatic aspects 28
    stress-mediated, neuromodulators 32
  excessive bleeding
    clinician inquiry 27
    psychosocial dynamics 27
  hormonal secretions 14
  luteal phase 14
  psychogenic disorders 29
Menstrual molimina 5
Midwifery 96
Mitosis 7
  granulosa cells 8, 11
Muscle relaxation hypnosis, cancer chemotherapy 161

Naloxone 31
Natural childbirth 101, 102
Neurohormones
  hypothalamic feedback 16
  secretion, anterior pituitary, retrograde blood flow 16
  synthesis and transport 17
  see also Thyrotropin-releasing hormone; Gonadotropin-releasing hormone
Neurons
  dopaminergic 20
  GnRH-secreting fibers 17
  norepinephrine 20
  neurohormone/neurotransmitter synthesis 17
Neurosecretion 15
Neurotransmitter
  hypothalamic feedback 16
  see also Biogenic amines
Norepinephrine
  GnRH release 29
  hypothalamic neurotransmitter 16
  midcycle LH surge 30

Oocyte
  growth 8, 9
  maturation-inhibitory factor (MIF) 13
  number, birth/puberty 35
  ovulation and atresia 36
  primary 7

Oogenesis 35
Oophorectomy 36
Opiates, endogenous 5, 21
Osteoporosis
  fractures 41
  pathogenic factors 40
  therapy 48
Ovarian function
  emotional stress 29
  failure, treatment 48
Ovary, follicle
  atresia, site 10
  dominant 21
  estrogen:androgen ratio 10
  secretion 5, 6
  fluid accumulation
    composition 9, 10
  growth stages 8–10
  maturation cessation 35, 36
  preovulatory selection 10
  primary, theca interna 8
  primordial 8
    atresia 7, 10
  secondary 9, 10
  wall rupture 10
    ovum extrusion 13
Ovulation
  cessation 7
  control 15, 20
  cycle
    factors affecting 5
    follicular phase 5–10, 35, 36
    hormonal events 5–7
    LH surge 6, 12
    luteal phase 9
    neuroendocrinology 5
    neurohormones 16
  endocrinology 2
  failure 12
  occurrence 13
  suppression 30

Pain
  components 124
  concepts 125, 126
  gynecologic causes 125
  labor/delivery, relaxation therapy 156

Subject Index

Pain (cont.)
  menstrual, treatment
    biofeedback 155
    group muscle training 154
  see also Pelvis; Pregnancy
Parental rights 177
Pelvis
  chronic pain 127, 128
  dependency needs 128
  depression, aspects 128, 130
  evaluation, medical 129, 130
  illness behavior 127
  management
    behavioral problems, options 132
    new methods 133, 134
    trials of therapy 132
  operant conditioning behavior 127, 128
Penis envy 60, 64
Perinatal care, emotional aspects 2
Phenethylamine (PEA), exercise-induced stress 30
Physician-patient relationships
  ethical principles 172–174
  inequality 169
  professional/moral responsibilities 171
  2-patient concept 167, 168
Pinocytosis 17
Pituitary
  anterior, nervous system influence 16
  gonadotropin secretion 5
  hypothalamus control 15
  LH release, pulsatile 18
  response to GnRH 5, 6
  sensitivity, pulsed GnRH ovulation control 15, 17, 18, 20–22
Placenta 31
Post-pill galactorrhea/amenorrhea 29
Pregnancy
  ambivalent attitudes 140
  childbirth
    fetal monitoring 96
    inclusion of men 98, 99
    preparatory classes 97
  corpus luteum progesterone 14
  high risk
    adolescents 82
    disease state attitude 72
  psychological impact 78
  nurturing role, spouse 77
  pain, behavioral therapy 157
  postpartum care 98
  psychological development
    adaptation 75, 76
    mothering role 73, 74
  stress
    amniocentesis 94, 99
    emotional 72, 74
    family 76
    fear of fetal loss 78
    hospitalization 78
    prenatal care 77
    specific responses 31
  ultrasound examination, value 95
Pregranulosa cells 8
Premenstrual changes 14
Premenstrual symptoms, depression/anger 154, 155
Prenatal care
  emotional aspects 2
  hormones, postnatal behavior 65
Preoedipal attachment 61
Preovulatory follicles 14
Progesterone
  corpus luteum secretion 14
  follicle growth 12, 13
  pregnancy 14, 15
  sequential therapy 48
  sexual drive 137
Progestin deficiency, endometrial hyperplasia 45
Progestogens 45
Prolactin
  dopamine effect 20
  hypersecretion 29, 30
    anovulation 31
  opioids 31
  secretion, sociopsychological distress 29
  TRH, influence 4
Proopiocortin 31
Prostaglandins 13, 15
Pseudocyesis 29, 32
Psyche-soma interdependence 2
Psychosexual response cycle
  Masters/Johnson concept 136

Subject Index

Psychosexual response cycle (cont.)
  sexual drive 136, 137
  tripartite, phases
    excitement 138
    orgasm, G-spot controversy 138
Psychosomatic medicine
  concepts 28
  facets of disease 27

Renin-angiotensin, aldosterone system 46
Reproduction
  basic concepts 2
  brain mechanisms 28
  endocrinology 28
  ethical issues 170
Retrograde axonal transport 16
Retrograde portal flow 16
Ribosome 17

Secondary sex changes 26
Serotonin 16
Sex hormone-binding globulin (SHBG) 17, 40
Sexism 169
Sexual response cycle
  concept 136
  tripartite phases 136, 137
Sexuality
  breast disease 144
  disease/distress patterns 136, 139
    psychological reaction, assessment 146
    tripartite scheme 147
  gynecologic malignancy 143, 144
  hysterectomy 142
  modifying factors 137, 138
  organic enjoyment 143
  postpartum 141
  pregnancy
    expectant father syndrome 141

  psychological factors 140, 141
  venereal disease 146
Sterilization, ethical issues 170, 171
Stress
  catecholamine formation 30
  hyperprolactinemia 31
  induced analgesia 31
  mediated events 30
  menses onset, 'honeymoon phenomenon' 32
  reproductive system 29
Surrogate mothers 176, 177
Systematic desensitization, dysmenorrhea 154

Testosterone
  postmenopause 37
  stress-mediated menstrual dysfunction 32
Theca cells 11–14
Theca interna 8, 10
Thromboembolic disease, oral contraceptives 47
Thrombophlebitis, estrogen replacement 47
Thyrotropin-releasing hormone (TRH)
  hypothalamic neurohormone 16
  pituitary prolactin 5
Tomboy behavior 65
Turner's syndrome 66

Vagina
  atrophy 42, 48
  core gender identity 61
  mental representation 60, 61
  orgasm 138
Vaginismus 157
Venereal disease 146

Women's Health Movement 166